BIOMEDICAL ETHICS

BIOMEDICAL ETHICS
A GUIDE TO DECISION MAKING

Robert T. Francoeur, Ph.D.

Professor of Allied Health Sciences
Fairleigh Dickinson University
Madison, New Jersey

A WILEY MEDICAL PUBLICATION
JOHN WILEY & SONS
New York • Chichester • Brisbane • Toronto • Singapore

Cover and interior design by Wanda Lubelska

Copyright © 1983 by John Wiley & Sons, Inc.

Library of Congress Cataloging in Publication Data:

Francoeur, Robert T.
  Biomedical ethics.

  (A Wiley medical publication)
  Includes index.
  1. Medical ethics—Addresses, essays, lectures.
I. Title. II. Series. [DNLM: 1. Ethics, Medical—
Programmed texts. 2. Decision making—Programmed
texts. W 50 F2855b]
R724.F65   1983   174'.2   83-6812
ISBN 0-471-09827-2

Printed in the United States of America

10 9 8 7 6 5 4 3 2 1

To Anna, my wife, and to our daughters, Nicole and Danielle, the silent partners in the creation of this text. Their combined love, patience, understanding, and, above all, Anna's pragmatic skepticism and sense of the real world, were key factors in the birth of this worktext.

PREFACE

Moral dilemmas abound today, especially in the area of health care. Newspapers, magazines, radio, and television daily highlight ethical issues in nuclear warfare, abortion, the right to refuse treatment, mercy killing, computerized medical records, human experimentation, informed consent, caring for the aged, equitable distribution of scarce resources, responsibility for environmental pollution, overpopulation, and many other issues. The existence of heated public debate on these topics is evidence that people have very different views of what is a morally "right" or "wrong" action. The sophistication of health care today has expanded and complicated the ethical dilemmas we face as we decide what are the moral rights and responsibilities of health care workers and their patients.

In addition, our sophisticated technologies have created new moral dilemmas never faced in the past. We know, for instance, that abortion has been *legally* right since the Supreme Court decision of 1973. The majority of Americans accept that it is *socially* right for a woman to have an abortion. An early abortion is a safe procedure and is therefore *medically* right, if the patient so decides. But answering questions about what is legally, socially, or medically right does not answer the question of what is *morally* right or wrong about abortion. In *Biomedical Ethics: A Guide to Decision Making* we focus on the practical steps used to make ethical or moral decisions.

This worktext is divided into two parts. Part One contains 16 chapters with information about the four levels of ethical thinking: systems, principles, values, and judgments or methods used in making ethical decisions. (See the schematic preview of the text following the Contents.) Part Two contains 16 chapters that parallel those in Part One. They provide you with the exercise pages for completing class assignments and applying the skills and techniques learned in Part One.

Thirty-five ethical dilemmas or brief case studies are used to illustrate the decision-making processes in Part One. A few of these cases are practical, everyday situations in the health care professions. More cases deal with unusual situations that have been national news. A few cases are "mind stretchers," futuristic cases that we need to consider as they are likely to become problems in 5 or 10 years.

The wide range of case studies chosen touches on all major ethical issues in health care today, but the cases themselves and the conclusions you reach with them are less important than reaching the two goals of (1) developing sensitivity to ethical issues and (2) mastering and understanding different ways in which decisions can be made. These practical decision-making skills can then be used in any situation encountered. No one can predict the particular ethical dilemmas you will face in the future, but if you have developed your skills in making ethical decisions, you will be better prepared to handle whatever dilemma you encounter.

A Brief Outline of This Worktext

The chapters in Part One are divided into three sections: Section I deals with ethical systems and our moral development; Section II deals with ethical principles and rules; and Section III provides specific decision-making exercises.

In Section I we look first at where we derive our sense of what is morally "right" and "wrong." Each of us grows up in a particular social environment in which influences, views, and information constantly mold our outlook and judgments of what we consider morally right or wrong. As infants, we do not know what is right and wrong. From our parents, our families, and other social interactions we soon become sensitive to different views about what is the right thing to do. Gradually we develop a personal sense of morality. In Chapter 1, we examine two basic world views and their relationship to two general ethical systems, one that focuses on moral duties and one that is concerned about the moral consequences of actions. In Chapter 2, we examine three theories of the stages we pass through as we develop a mature sensitivity to moral issues. These theories suggest that men and women initially have quite different approaches to ethical dilemmas and judgments. We need to become sensitive to how our world view, the basic ethical system we follow, and our social conditioning as male or female influence our ethical decisions.

Section II contains two chapters. The first is an exercise in identifying ethical principles, especially in professional codes of ethical conduct. The second is an exercise in identifying and sorting out the ethical values or rules that we derive from our ethical principles in particular cases.

The 12 chapters in Section III of Part One illustrate different methods you can use in making ethical decisions. Chapter 5 is an exercise in deciding who should be treated when there is a shortage of equipment or other resources. Chapter 6 examines the ethical responsibilities and rights of the patient and health care worker that result from the implied contract they enter into. In Chapter 7 you are asked to identify and sort all the options or alternatives that might be found in a situation. You need to know what your options are before you can make a reasonable choice.

Chapters 8, 9, 10, and 11 illustrate the use of an operational decision, a decisional balance sheet focusing on costs and benefits for your best options, a decision tree, and the quantitative approach of a decision matrix. Chapter 12 creates a situation in which you cope with the least desirable option. In Chapters 13 and 14 you explore the influence on your ethical decision of personal motives and the way a case is presented. Suggestions are given in Chapter 15 for reaching a decision on an ethical dilemma using the jury or committee approach. Chapter 16 focuses on the central and ultimate question behind all ethical problems: Who is a person? To begin to answer it, we must also ask, why do we attribute to someone personhood and human rights, and when do we achieve and lose that status?

Using This Worktext and Its Exercises

Biomedical ethics focuses on moral judgments applied to the delivery of health care. In this worktext, we have two goals: (1) improving your sensitivity to ethical issues in health care, and (2) developing your decision-making skills. Making decisions is never easy. The moral dilemmas outlined in this worktext, and those you encounter in your clinical experience, will never be easy to resolve. Solutions are seldom immediately obvious.

If you are using this worktext in a course, your instructor will schedule the sequence of chapters and exercises. After a chapter has been explained and illustrated with a sample case in class, you may be asked to complete the accompanying exercise in Part Two as homework. These exercises may also be used as tests or as practice sheets. Some or all of your exercises may be graded and used as one element in determining your course grade.

If you are using this worktext on your own for professional or personal enrichment, set your own pace. Read a chapter and think about it. Pick another case or situation that interests you, perhaps one you encountered in your clinical work or one you heard from others or read about in the news. Work the case through with the appropriate blank form in Part Two.

The exercises and methods illustrated in Part One and available for your own use with a second case in Part Two may at times appear overly detailed and too mechanical. However, by breaking down the process of decision making and by analyzing each step in different methods, you will appreciate the process of making good decisions. To aid in the analysis, each exercise is divided into several phases.

Take your time in thinking through each step in the exercise before you begin to write. Do not waste limited space on irrelevant ideas or poorly thought out reasons. The care and analysis you put into the decision-making process are more important than your conclusion.

As stated above, this is a worktext whose focus and goals are to help you become more sensitive to ethical dilemmas in health care and more skilled in making good ethical decisions. One of the best ways to appreciate and learn the sensitivity and skills that are part of making good ethical decisions in medical situations is to practice these various methods on your own. Then when you encounter new situations and problems you will naturally apply the skills you have acquired without having to go through a particular method as you do here. The skills will carry over into everyday situations and decisions. The result will be health care that is more humane and holistic and that respects the dignity and integrity of both the consumer and the health care worker.

Robert T. Francoeur

ACKNOWLEDGMENTS

Special acknowledgment is paid to Ruth Elsasser, Professor Emerita and past Allied Health Program Administrator at Fairleigh Dickinson University, Madison, New Jersey. It was with the strong support and encouragement from this dear friend and colleague that I began, in 1972, to teach biomedical ethics to students in our new Allied Health Program under a Department of Health, Education, and Welfare grant she designed.

For clinical input and evaluation I thank Barbara Lee Picorale, R.T., (R)C.X.T., Allied Health Professor and Radiologic Technology Program Director, Morristown Memorial Hospital, Morristown, New Jersey; David Bloom, M.D., Medical Director, Radiology, Morristown Memorial Hospital; Virginia Bertholf, M.A., R.P.T., Allied Health Professor and Physical Therapy Program Director, Morristown Memorial Hospital; Nicholas Sconzo, R.R.T., Director of Respiratory Therapy Program, St. Clare's Hospital, Denville, New Jersey; David Lasco, R.R.T., Allied Health Associate Professor and Respiratory Therapy Program Director, St. Clare's Hospital; Allan Stein, M.D., Director of Rehabilitation Medicine, Beth Israel Medical Center, Newark, New Jersey; James F. Whitacre, M.S., R.R.T., School of Health Related Professions, The University of Missouri at Columbia.

For critical input from allied health educators I thank Joseph Hamburg, M.D., Dean, College of Allied Health Professions, The University of Kentucky, Lexington, Kentucky; Edmund McTernan, Ed.D., Dean, School of Allied Health Professions, State University of New York at Stony Brook; Roger Marion, Ph.D., School of Allied Health Sciences, The University of Texas Medical Branch at Galveston; Thomas McElhinney, Ph.D., Chairman of General Studies, School of Allied Health, Thomas Jefferson School of Medicine, Philadelphia; Marion Kayhart, Ph.D., Chairman of Biology, Cedar Crest College, Allentown, Pennsylvania; Joseph Fletcher, Visiting Professor of Medical Ethics, The University of Virginia School of Medicine at Richmond and The Texas Medical Center at Galveston.

Others who provided input and critical evaluations were Mona L. Fiorentini, M.H.A., Director of Planning and Marketing, Memorial General Hospital, Union, New Jersey; Byron Lambert, Professor of Philosophy and Ethics, Fairleigh Dickinson University, Madison, New Jersey; Linda Hendrixson, New York University Health Education Program; Stephen Wang, M.D., Director of Medical Education, Morristown Memorial Hospital; George Sellmer, Ph.D., Upsala College, East Orange, New Jersey; Ellen Dupont and Robert Milford, Fairleigh Dickinson University.

Robert T. Francoeur

CONTENTS

PART TWO: EXERCISES AND FORMS FOR APPLYING DECISION-MAKING STEPS AND TECHNIQUES

BIOMEDICAL ETHICS

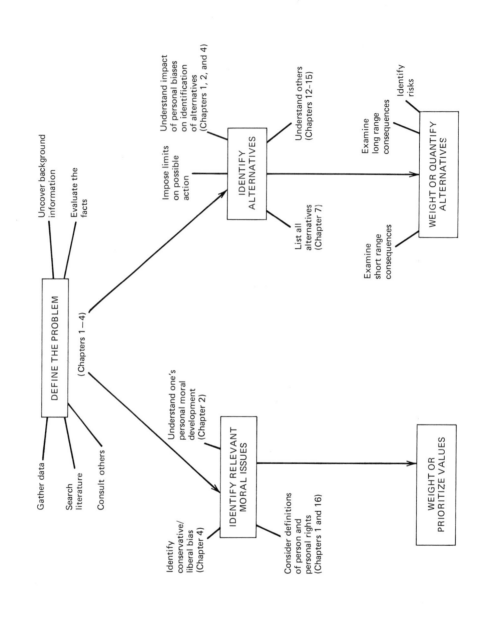

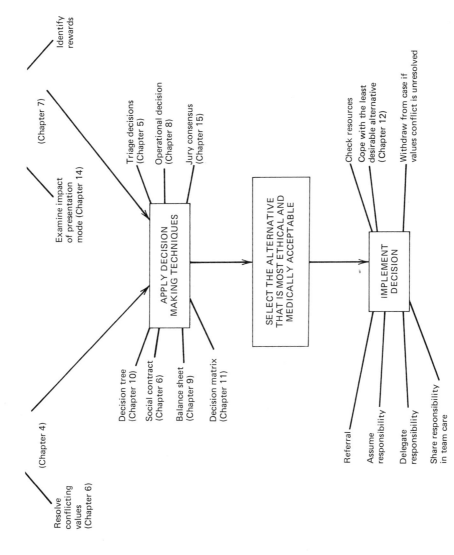

Identify
rewards

(Chapter 7)

Examine impact
of presentation
mode (Chapter 14)

Triage decisions
(Chapter 5)

Operational decision
(Chapter 8)

Jury consensus
(Chapter 15)

Check resources

Cope with the least
desirable alternative
(Chapter 12)

Withdraw from case if
values conflict is unresolved

(Chapter 4)

APPLY DECISION
MAKING TECHNIQUES

SELECT THE ALTERNATIVE
THAT IS MOST ETHICAL AND
MEDICALLY ACCEPTABLE

IMPLEMENT
DECISION

Resolve
conflicting
values
(Chapter 6)

Decision tree
(Chapter 10)

Social contract
(Chapter 6)

Balance sheet
(Chapter 9)

Decision matrix
(Chapter 11)

Referral

Assume
responsibility

Delegate
responsibility

Share responsibility
in team care

Preview of the text. This schema of the decision-making process is adapted to the issues of biomedical ethics. The chapters that discuss the specific steps are indicated in parentheses.

(Adapted from Hill, P., et al. *Making Decisions: A Multidisciplinary Introduction.* Reading, MA: Addison-Wesley, 1978, p. 22. Reprinted with permission.)

PART ONE
A GUIDE TO INDIVIDUAL STEPS AND TECHNIQUES IN DECISION MAKING

Section I
Ethical Systems and Moral Development

1

TWO WORLD VIEWS AND TWO ASSOCIATED VALUE SYSTEMS

CHAPTER 1

TWO WORLD VIEWS
AND TWO ASSOCIATED
VALUE SYSTEMS

In this chapter there are two questions we need to examine. First, we want to know what are the basic ethical systems from which people derive their conclusions about what is right and wrong? Second, we want to find out where do these different ethical systems come from? Are there different ways of looking at the world we live in that can lead people to such opposing views of abortion, nuclear war, or capital punishment? Abortion, in fact, is an excellent example for us to use in answering these two questions. It is likely to be a subject on which you have strong opinions and on which others have equally strong, if different, positions. These different positions can serve as an example of two basic world views and of two general ethical systems derived from those views.

A Specific Ethical Issue: Abortion

Abortion is condemned by the Right To Life movement, by Protestant ethicists such as Paul Ramsey at Princeton Theological Seminary, by the Moral Majority, by some voters, and by some of our elected representatives, including President Ronald Reagan and Senators Orrin Hatch, Mark Hatfield, Jesse Helms, and Henry Hyde, who strongly support antiabortion legislation. It is condemned by the Vatican, by the Eastern Orthodox Church, and by other churches. These quite different groups all share a common *absolutist view* of human life and ethics. For them, human life comes into existence as an absolute complete entity at the particular moment when the egg and sperm unite or when the fertilized egg implants in the lining of the uterus. From that moment on, the tiny embryonic mass enjoys the same rights as any other person. From some specific time very early in embryonic life until absolute death, all human beings share the same equal absolute sacred right to life without any possibility of compromise. The first diagram in Figure 1.1 illustrates this ethical position and suggests

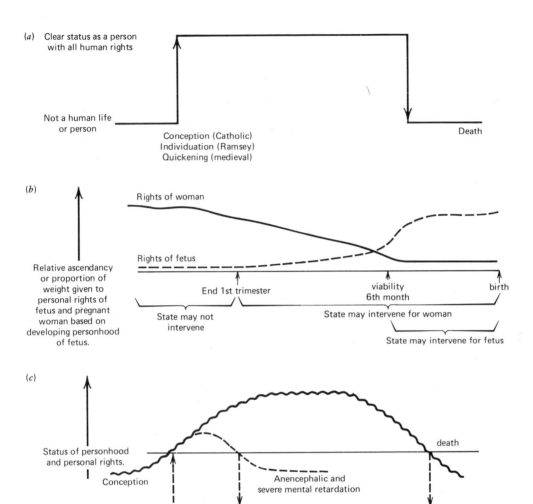

(a) Clear status as a person with all human rights

Not a human life or person

Conception (Catholic)
Individuation (Ramsey)
Quickening (medieval)

Death

(b)

Rights of woman

Rights of fetus

Relative ascendancy or proportion of weight given to personal rights of fetus and pregnant woman based on developing personhood of fetus.

End 1st trimester

viability
6th month

birth

State may not intervene

State may intervene for woman

State may intervene for fetus

(c)

Status of personhood and personal rights.

death

Conception

Anencephalic and severe mental retardation

FIGURE 1.1 *Three philosophical or legal positions on abortion. (**a**) The antiabortion position is often based on a fixed philosophy of nature and an absolutist world view in which human personhood is an all-or-nothing quantity. This status comes into existence at conception, individuation, or some specific point, and ceases at a second point in time. One either has all the rights of a person or does not enjoy status as a human. (**b**) The legal position of the U.S. Supreme Court tries to balance the rights of the fetus as they emerge over a 9-month pregnancy with the full personhood status of the pregnant woman. The balance shifts in favor of the personal rights of the fetus as it reaches term. This view is based on a process world view. (**c**) The third position is also based on a developmental or process world view but focuses on the emerging personhood and personal rights of the fetus before and after birth. The exact determination of when personhood status begins or ends and its relative quality depends on the criteria selected.*

(Drawings and explanation adapted from Brody, H. *Ethical Decisions in Medicine*, 2nd ed. Boston: Little, Brown, 1981. Used with permission.)

comparison with the two other views shown in the second and third diagrams of the same figure.

On the opposite side of this debate are advocates of freedom of choice, the U.S. Supreme Court, Catholics for Free Choice, the Religious Coalition for Abortion Rights, Planned Parenthood, the National Organization for Women, and others. This ethical position is based on a *process view* rather than on an absolutist view of human nature. Following the lead of the Supreme Court in its 1973 decision that gave women the legal right to have an abortion, the advocates of freedom of choice argue that we must recognize the rights of two human beings in this situation. Under the Fourteenth Amendment a woman should have the right to control her own body. At the same time a new human being is coming into existence in her uterus. We also have to respect the growing rights of the developing fetus. Instead of picking a specific point in time, for the embryonic mass suddenly to be endowed with full absolute human rights, such as fertilization or conception, this second position tries to balance the rights of the woman and those of the developing fetus. Instead of an all-or-nothing view of human life, this view emphasizes the development of "personhood" and the variability in the "quality of human life." In this view, the rights of the developing embryo gradually gain equality with and, in the third trimester of pregnancy, take priority over the woman's control over her body. The middle diagram in Figure 1.1 shows this legal position.

The decision of the U.S. Supreme Court is a legal interpretation of a philosophical and ethical approach to human nature that emphasizes the developmental processes from fertilization to the grave. This approach considers human life in terms of its quality rather than as an all-or-nothing "quantity." This raises a heated debate about what criteria we select to define "personhood." If we decide that cerebral cortical activity is the essential criterion, then, until the embryo actually exercises this capacity, it is not a person and does not have the right to life, although its potential personal rights do deserve respect. The coma victim diagnosed as brain dead may also not be considered a person, although he or she still has human life. The quality of life makes a discussion of criteria for personhood crucial, but our scientific understanding is still too primitive in the areas of developmental psychology, neurophysiology, and neuroanatomy for us to agree on valid criteria for personhood. (The problem of defining personhood will be the focus of our last chapter.)

For the moment, if you compare the third diagram in Figure 1.1 with the first diagram, you will see that this process view individualizes every situation and decision. It raises questions of personhood and of the relative weight and merit of the personal rights of the pregnant woman and the fetus she is carrying. It arises with the anencephalic infant, with the severely mentally retarded, and with the comatose patient with severe irreversible brain damage.

Two Ethical Systems—Two World Views

Ernst Mayr, a Harvard biologist, a philosopher, and the author of *Animal Species and Evolution*, once noted that since earliest human history there have been two opposing ways of looking at the world. One view has emphasized an unchanging world of absolutes created in the beginning of time. The other view emphasizes variation and individuality in an ever-changing world and developing human nature. "No two ways of looking at Nature could be more different," wrote Mayr in 1963.

The history of philosophy makes it clear that every human effort at creating a theology, a philosophy, or an ethical system starts with the way the individual or the group pictures the world. Our ethical systems, on which we base our judgments of abortion and other moral problems, grow out of our particular *weltanschauung*, or world view.

Some people view the world as a completely finished universe with human nature created perfect and complete in the beginning. In the Christian tradition, the story of Genesis explains our present imperfect world as a fall from divine grace, but human nature remains complete in its essence. Human nature, then, is an all-or-nothing absolute, a total entity that is or is not, with no gray zones. Out of this world view come a variety of ethical systems that we will cluster under the general title of *duty-oriented ethical systems*. In the professional literature, the most common label for these systems is "deontological," from *deon*, the Greek word for "duty," and *logos*, the Greek word for "discourse." Other system labels used are "absolutist," "formalist," and "Kantian imperatives." Individuals in this broad tradition might call themselves "Oxford intuitionists," "contract theorists," or "nonconsequentialists."

Four main schools of ethical thought can be grouped under the duty-oriented category. The oldest schools in this tradition are the Hebrew-Christian and Moslem ethics which conceive the ideal moral life as obedience to the will of God and the positive laws or rules that express the divine will. Likewise, Immanuel Kant's ethics also focus on duty, holding that the requirements of morality always override all other reasons for acting. Two of Kant's themes are quite compatible with the Hebrew-Christian ethic: (1) the ideal life consists in submitting our judgment to certain universal imperatives that bind everyone without exception; and (2) moral imperatives are unconditional, absolute, supreme, and universal. Kant's last two conclusions, however, are incompatible with the Hebrew-Christian ethic: (3) the authority that the morally good person submits to is not an outside authority but the rational logic of one's own will; and (4) certain liberal values must be respected, including autonomy, freedom, dignity, self-respect, and respect for individual rights.

The Oxford Intuitionists believe that the moral rightness or wrongness of an act depends on its intrinsic nature. Intrinsic in every act are certain elements that make it right or wrong. These can be known by intuition and need to be weighed and balanced against each other before one can be certain what is the moral course of action. The fourth duty-oriented school is that established by John Rawls, who emphasizes the obligations of justice that bind every human in a contractual relationship.

For the duty-oriented ethicists, the absoluteness of right and wrong can reside in *rules* and principles or in the intrinsic rightness or wrongness of particular *acts* known intuitively (Fig. 1.2).

On the other end of the spectrum of ethical systems are what we call the *consequence-oriented ethical systems*. These include ethical systems known as "teleological" because they focus on the outcome of our actions, "consequentialist" because of a focus on consequences, "utilitarian," "situation ethics," and "egoist ethics."

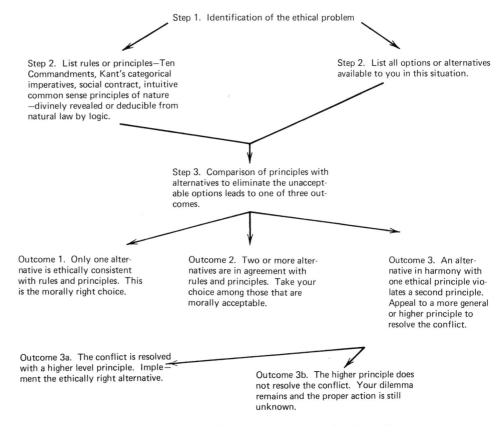

Step 1. Identification of the ethical problem

Step 2. List rules or principles—Ten Commandments, Kant's categorical imperatives, social contract, intuitive common sense principles of nature —divinely revealed or deducible from natural law by logic.

Step 2. List all options or alternatives available to you in this situation.

Step 3. Comparison of principles with alternatives to eliminate the unacceptable options leads to one of three outcomes.

Outcome 1. Only one alternative is ethically consistent with rules and principles. This is the morally right choice.

Outcome 2. Two or more alternatives are in agreement with rules and principles. Take your choice among those that are morally acceptable.

Outcome 3. An alternative in harmony with one ethical principle violates a second principle. Appeal to a more general or higher principle to resolve the conflict.

Outcome 3a. The conflict is resolved with a higher level principle. Implement the ethically right alternative.

Outcome 3b. The higher principle does not resolve the conflict. Your dilemma remains and the proper action is still unknown.

FIGURE 1.2 *Flow chart showing the duty-oriented process of making ethical decisions.*

(Adapted from Brody, H. *Ethical Decisions in Medicine,* 2nd ed. Boston: Little, Brown, 1981. Used with permission.)

In the view of some ethicists, the duty-oriented and the consequence-oriented systems are mutually exclusive, whereas for others they represent convenient labels for interestingly different but not mutually exclusive ethical systems. Because of the overlap in this spectrum and the existence of ethical systems that are a mixture of both duty and consequence orientations, we will use the terms *duty-oriented* and *consequence-oriented* in a nonexclusive sense as general but not absolute labels.

As with the duty-oriented ethicists, we have *act consequence-oriented theories* that use a basic principle of promoting the most good for the most people in particular acts in particular circumstances. *Rule consequence-oriented theories* apply the same principle of the greatest good for the most people to general rules of conduct, which then tell us whether our acts are right or wrong.

Consequence-oriented ethical systems are deeply rooted in a process view, just as duty-oriented ethical systems are more inclined to the absolutist world view. Both the world and human nature are in the process of evolving and developing (Fig. 1.3).

Despite the close link between duty-oriented ethics and absolutist world views, and between consequence-oriented ethics and an evolutionary world view, the dichotomy is often blurred when specific ethical issues are considered. People may take an absolutist duty-oriented position in one situation and then apply

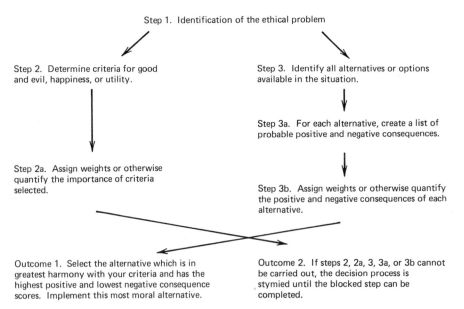

Step 1. Identification of the ethical problem

Step 2. Determine criteria for good and evil, happiness, or utility.

Step 3. Identify all alternatives or options available in the situation.

Step 3a. For each alternative, create a list of probable positive and negative consequences.

Step 2a. Assign weights or otherwise quantify the importance of criteria selected.

Step 3b. Assign weights or otherwise quantify the positive and negative consequences of each alternative.

Outcome 1. Select the alternative which is in greatest harmony with your criteria and has the highest positive and lowest negative consequence scores. Implement this most moral alternative.

Outcome 2. If steps 2, 2a, 3, 3a, or 3b cannot be carried out, the decision process is stymied until the blocked step can be completed.

FIGURE 1.3 *Flow chart showing the consequence-oriented process of making ethical decisions.*

(Adapted from Brody, H. *Ethical Decisions in Medicine.* Boston: Little, Brown, 1981. Used with permission.)

a consequence-oriented view to a second problem. It is interesting to note the persistency of these two systems. You find both in every religious tradition and in many cultures. Table 1.1 attempts to display the range of ethical thought in different religious traditions and to relate these different ethical views in terms of their basic cosmological and philosophical outlooks. There is often more agreement among different groups on the right or left side of the spectrum than there is among persons at opposite ends of the spectrum within a particular religious tradition. Protestants in the covenant tradition on the right side, for instance, have more in common with the liberal process-oriented Catholic theologians than they do with their Protestant fundamentalist brethren. The Moslem world in Iran, Iraq, Egypt, and Pakistan has been racked by conflicts and violence between duty-oriented fundamentalists and other Moslems who are willing to adapt their traditions to the needs of a rapidly changing industrial world.*

TABLE 1.1   Spectrum of Ethical Systems and Their Interrelationships

	Continuum or Spectrum	
World view or cosmology	Fixed philosophy of nature	Process philosophy of nature
Ethical system	Duty-oriented ethics	Consequence-oriented or covenant ethics
Tradition		
Protestant	Biblical literal fundamentalism, Moral Majority	Covenant tradition in Presbyterian, Methodist churches; Episcopal process theologians
Judaic	Hassidic concern for strict observance of the Torah and talmudic prescriptions	Liberal or reformed application of moral principles to today's situations
Roman Catholic	Static, act-oriented; ethics based on the natural law and the Divine Order	Evolutionary, process- and person-oriented ethic
Moslem	Concern for literal interpretation of the Koran and return to the purity of early Islam; fundamentalist	Ethics and culture emphasizing need for adapting the Koran to modern Western life and technological advances
Humanist	Stoicism and epicurean asceticism	Situation ethics

*Some of the dimensions for this comparison were suggested by Richard Kropf, S.T.M., Ph.D.

Some ethicists who focus on the consequences of rules come close to some more liberal, duty-oriented ethicists of the natural law tradition. The contract ethics of John Rawls, for instance, are a widely acclaimed mix of Kant's natural imperatives and Joseph Fletcher's situation ethics. In Rawls' theory of justice the idea of a covenant or social contract between the moral agents is the crucial factor. When free and rational persons enter into an implied or explicit contract as part of their relationships, they should be choosing principles of justice that advance the good of society's members. These principles not only determine what actions are right or wrong in the context of the relationship and of society, but they also determine personal and social rights and the distribution of benefits and burdens within the society. It is in this latter area of balancing the benefits and burdens of society that Rawls' theory may prove helpful in the years ahead.

The recent trend toward convergence of duty- and consequence-oriented schools can be illustrated by a practical issue, that of the confidentiality required between the health care professional and the patient. Both consequence-oriented and duty-oriented ethicists can defend the need for absolute confidentiality. However, in certain circumstances, when the harmful consequences or a principle of higher social good require, both approaches may defend the breaking of patient confidentiality.

Once a person chooses his or her basic world view, then everything else in their outlook on life, their values, and their behavior seems to be colored by this basic world view, including their conclusions about issues in medical ethics.

Professional Confidentiality Viewed From the Perspective of Different Ethical Systems

Now that we have examined the two basic world views of finished and evolving natures, and the duty-oriented and consequences-oriented general ethical systems that are derived from these two world views, we can apply these perspectives to a case study in which using the two systems can lead to different conclusions about what is the more ethical way to act.

In August 1969, Prosenjiit Poddar, a young voluntary out-patient being treated at the University of California at Berkeley, informed his psychologist that he was going to kill an unidentified woman. From working with the young man, the psychologist knew who the woman was. After consulting with his superior and a psychiatrist, the psychologist asked the campus police to detain Prosenjiit so he could be committed to a mental hospital for observation. The police took Prosenjiit into custody, but soon released him when he appeared rational. The psychologist's superior then withdrew and destroyed all written letters and notes, and ordered no further action to commit Prosenjiit. No one warned the woman, although she was expected to return to Berkeley soon.

Shortly afterward, Prosenjiit persuaded the woman's brother to share an apartment with him near where she lived with her parents. Later, Prosenjiit visited the young woman and killed her.

When the murdered woman's parents learned that the psychologist, two consultants, and the police had known of Prosenjiit's threats, they sued in court. They charged that these parties were criminally negligent in permitting Prosenjiit to be released from police custody without notifying them or their daughter of the danger she was in (Beauchamp & Childress, 1979, pp. 246–250).

What was the ethical responsibility of the psychologist in this case? Should he have warned the woman of her danger? Or was his primary and sole obligation to respect the confidentiality of the information he gained during his treatment of Prosenjiit? Is patient confidentiality an absolute rule, with no exceptions? Or, are there some circumstances when the psychologist, health care professional, or other professional may disclose information that comes to him or her as part of a patient's treatment? And if so, what are these circumstances? Might preserving the welfare of an innocent third person, or of society, serve as a higher absolute duty than the duty to maintain patient confidentiality? What are the consequences of allowing exceptions?

You can approach this case from a duty-oriented ethic. If you accept as an absolute moral obligation the guidelines of the World Medical Association International Code of Medical Ethics, you would conclude that the psychologist and others in this case owe the patient "absolute secrecy on all [information] which has been confided to him or which he knows because of the confidence entrusted to him."

But you might also come to the same conclusion from the viewpoint of a consequence orientation focusing on the social harm that would result from violating the rule of the World Medical Association on confidentiality just cited. The judge who dissented from the majority opinion in this case argued that the obligation to confidentiality is primary and near-absolute, not because of some principle or rule, but because "overwhelming policy considerations weigh against imposing a duty on psychotherapists to warn a potential victim against harm." The dissenting judge cited three reasons based on consequences for holding that the obligation of confidentiality prohibited the psychologist in this case from revealing his knowledge to anyone, even the police: "While offering virtually no benefit to society, such a duty will frustrate psychiatric treatment, invade fundamental patient rights, and increase violence." These three harmful social consequences far outweighed the possible benefits to one person.

On the opposite side, most codes of medical and professional ethics hold that the rule of confidentiality is not absolute. The American Medical Association code, for instance, holds that a "physician may not reveal the confidences entrusted to him in the course of medical attendance, or the deficiencies he may observe in the character of his patients, unless he is required to do so by law or unless it becomes necessary in order to protect the welfare of the individual or of the community." The social good or protection of an innocent third party can be cited as a higher duty. Or, changing the perspective slightly, relative confidentiality can be viewed as contributing to the good of society and innocent persons.

In the court case of Prosenjiit, the majority opinion of the judges followed the qualified rule of the American Medical Association. The majority opinion held that two ethical obligations were in conflict, the obligation to protect the confidentiality of the patient and the obligation to protect innocent persons from violence and possible death. Weighing the possible harm to the patient in breaking confidentiality and the benefit to the young woman, the majority held that the moral obligation of confidentiality was less important than the obligation to protect an innocent party.

In this case, and in most other cases encountered in biomedical ethics, one can come to quite different solutions depending on the ethical system followed and the interpretations of that ethical system and its principles.

Applying This Approach to Your Case Study

In Part Two of this worktext you will find exercise pages for this chapter. You can use these pages to help sharpen your understanding of the two basic ethical systems and how they work. Using a case of your own choice or one assigned to you, identify two opposing solutions based on a general principle of morality. Then, following the general outline of duty-oriented and consequence-oriented reasonings given in the sample case above and in Figures 1.2 and 1.3, develop arguments to support and defend these different solutions.

REFERENCES AND FURTHER READINGS

Barry, V. *Moral Aspects of Health Care.* Belmont, CA: Wadsworth, 1982, pp. 59–90.

Beauchamp, T.L., & Childress, J.F. *Principles of Biomedical Ethics.* New York: Oxford University Press, 1979.

Beauchamp, T.L., & Walters, L. *Contemporary Issues in Bioethics.* Belmont, CA: Wadsworth, 1982, pp. 7–26, 204–211.

Francoeur, R.T. *Perspectives in Evolution.* Baltimore: Helicon, 1965.

Francoeur, R.T. *Evolving World Converging Man.* New York: Holt Rinehart & Winston, 1970.

Harron, F., Burnside, J., & Beauchamp, T. *Health Care and Human Values: A Guide to Making Your Own Decisions.* New Haven: Yale University Press, 1983.

Kieffer, G.H. *Bioethics: A Textbook of Issues.* Reading, MA: Addison-Wesley, 1979, pp. 51–61.

Mayr, E. *Animal Species and Evolution.* Cambridge, MA: Harvard Belknap, 1963.

Munson, R. *Intervention and Reflection: Basic Issues in Medical Ethics,* 2nd ed. Belmont, CA: Wadsworth, 1983, pp. 1–40.

Pence, G.E. *Ethical Options in Medicine.* Oradell, NJ: Medical Economics, 1980, pp. 21–52.

Rawls, J. *A Theory of Justice.* Cambridge, MA: Harvard University Press, 1971.

Reich, W.T., ed. *The Encyclopedia of Bioethics.* New York: Free Press/Collier Macmillan, 1978, pp. 413–437.

2   THREE MODELS
OF MORAL DEVELOPMENT

CHAPTER 2
THREE MODELS
OF MORAL DEVELOPMENT

We are born without a conscious sense of morality or ethics, whatever intuitive or natural base of moral principles one might claim exists. As infants we do not understand the difference between good and evil actions. We learn this distinction only gradually as we are conditioned by our parents, society, and other factors in our environment. Part of this conditioning involves the ways we learn to view the world in fixed or process terms and the relative stress we learn to give duty and consequences. Another important aspect, which is considered in this chapter, is the possible effect of our gender and the social condition associated with it. Together these three factors very much influence what behaviors we find either acceptable or unacceptable, good or evil.

Three theories of moral development, discussed in this chapter, have been proposed to explain the stages through which we pass as we become morally sensitive. As such, they are important to keep in mind as we examine the various methods of making decisions about biomedical ethics.

Initially, we need to be aware of two important limitations. The first two models, those proposed by Jean Piaget and Lawrence Kohlberg, are attractive because of their precise logic and structured sequence of steps. However, both of these models are exclusively derived from research with boys. They analyze moral development in terms of male experiences and assume that male experiences are the norm for moral maturity. Our third model, proposed recently by Carol Gilligan, does not have the strength of Kohlberg's and Piaget's longitudinal studies nor does it have their structure and sequential steps. It does, however, add an important new dimension to our thinking by challenging the male bias of the other models and bringing to light a different, equally mature sense of morality evident in the female experience. The real meaning of these brief cautionary notes will become evident as we examine the three theories (Table 2.1).

Piaget's Theory of Moral Development

One of the most respected of modern psychologists, Jean Piaget (1896–1980) is well known for his work in developmental psychology. In suggesting a model to explain our growth as moral persons, Piaget was quick to stress that moral

TABLE 2.1 Comparison of the Stages in Two Models of Moral Development as Proposed by Jean Piaget and Lawrence Kohlberg

Piaget's Moral Development Model	Kohlberg's Moral Development Model			
	Level	Orientation Stage	Characterized by:	Personally Stated as:
Amoral stage—ages 0 to 2				
Egocentric stage—ages 2 to 7—lacks morality, bends rules, and reacts instinctively to environment	Preconventional	1. Punishment and obedience orientation	Total respect for authority	I must obey the authority figure, or else . . .
		2. Instrumental relativist orientation	Satisfying one's own needs	I might if I want to, but don't count on it.
Heteronomous stage—ages 7 to 12—based on total acceptance of a morality imposed by others	Conventional	3. Good boy– nice girl orientation	Conformity to social conventions and expectations	I probably should because everyone expects me to.
		4. Law and order orientation	Respect for authority and society's laws	I ought to because of duty to obey the rules.
Autonomous stage—age 12 and over— based on an internalized morality of cooperation	Postconventional or autonomous	5. Social contract orientation	Conformity to the ever-changing values and demands of society	I may because of my role in society, but I often question the relative values of society.
		6. Universal ethical principle orientation	My conscience holds me responsible for doing what is right	I will because I know it is the right thing to do.

SOURCE: Francoeur, R.T. *Becoming a Sexual Person.* New York: John Wiley & Sons, 1982, p. 673.

development is intimately tied to the development of both cognitive (intellectualizing) and physical (motor–sensory) skills.

The infant, in Piaget's theory, begins life completely amoral, a totally self-centered being. Around age 2, the child enters the *egocentric stage*. Between ages 2 and 7, the child has only a very general idea of what rules are. He often changes the rules to satisfy his personal needs and whims, reacting instinctively to his environment with little moral sense.

The third level, which Piaget calls the *heteronomous stage,* is characterized by a morality of constraint. Under adult pressure, the child begins to exercise some degree of moral and logical control over his or her behavior. Between ages 7 and 12, the child learns to distinguish between valid and invalid ideas. Moral issues are seen in black and white terms, with outside authorities (parents, teachers, and older children) as the main factors in determining what is right or wrong. At this stage the emphasis is on a total acceptance of morality imposed by others, and therefore the understanding of real morality is limited.

As the child moves beyond the morality of heteronomy, he begins to comprehend values and to apply them in original ways. Some time after age 12, and continuing into adult life, the child enters a final level of moral sensitivity, the *autonomous stage.* This morality is characterized by cooperation rather than constraint. Interaction with peers, discussions, self-criticism, a sense of equality, and respect for others are major factors in this growth. Rules and ideas are questioned, tested, and verified. Those rules that are found to be morally acceptable are internalized, becoming an integral part of our personal morality.

In adolescence, Piaget observes, boys see rules in terms of peer agreement and what is judged to be mutually beneficial. Teenagers rebel against parental morality. Their moral judgments flip-flop. Yet in the end they often return to the morality they so vehemently rejected in their teen years.

Piaget makes a strong point about moral development being impossible without sufficient cognitive development. He adds the need for social interaction, but views this solely in terms of the boys he studied. Nothing is said about the quite different socialization and relationship patterns that girls experience.

Kohlberg's Theory of Moral Development

Lawrence Kohlberg's model of moral development is very similar to Piaget's, although it expands upon his in some new directions. Piaget's theory proposes four stages—amoral, egocentric, heteronomous, and autonomous—occurring generally at certain age breaks. Ignoring the amoral infant phase, Kohlberg's theory focuses on three levels—preconventional, conventional, and postconventional. He then divides each of these three levels into two stages.

On Kohlberg's *preconventional level,* the child responds to cultural rules and labels of good and bad. In the first of the two stages of this level, a total respect for authority rather than any respect for or understanding of morality directs one's behavior. In the second stage, behavior is motivated by satisfying one's own needs rather than by concern with the needs of others or of society.

Kohlberg's second level, the *conventional level,* is characterized by conforming to and maintaining the moral conventions expected by one's family, group, or culture, regardless of the personal consequences. In the "good boy–nice girl" stage of this level, the child conforms to social norms in order to win approval as "good" or "nice." In the second stage of the conventional level, the focus is on fixed rules, on respect for authority and law, and on maintaining the social order.

The third level proposed by Kohlberg, the *postconventional level,* occurs when the individual makes a clear effort to define his or her morality apart from outside authorities. In the "social contract" stage of this level the person sees himself or herself as a participant in a changing network of social obligations and responsibilities. Laws change to meet new social needs and the individual adapts to this change. In the sixth and highest stage of moral development, that of "universal ethical principles," abstract qualities such as justice, human rights, respect for the dignity of human life, and equality are important as one's conscience serves as the final judge in ethical dilemmas.

The similarities between the moral development models proposed by Piaget and Kohlberg are clearly evident in Table 2.1. On the far right of this table are some personal expressions that typify Kohlberg's six levels of moral development. We will use these statements in our exercise for this chapter. You might also ask yourself where the ethical systems mentioned in Chapter 1 fit into the Piaget and Kohlberg schemas. Would you classify Ramsey's duty-oriented and Kant's categorical imperative systems as preconventional, conventional, or postconventional; autonomous or heteronomous? Where does Rawls' social contract system fit in? What characteristics of the systems mentioned in Chapter 1 suggested your classification? As for cosmology or world view, which perspective, fixed or process, might Kohlberg and Piaget be more comfortable with in terms of their philosophical assumptions?

Gilligan's Theory of Moral Development

Both Piaget and Kohlberg describe moral maturity in terms of the male-dominated world of business. The sequence is logical, detailing an expansion in moral sensitivity and action from the individual to the societal to the universal principle level. Because his own needs dominate, the individual on the egocentric or preconventional level of moral development cannot see morality in terms of relations with others. On the conventional or heteronomous level, maintaining the existing norms of society is all important because these sustain relationships, families, and communities. On the sublime mature postconventional or autonomous level of moral development, the individual transcends utilitarian social concerns to base his morality on internalized universal principles and abstract values, especially that of justice.

Prominent among those who consistently appear deficient in moral development on these scales are women. Generally they seem to exemplify the conventional good boy–nice girl morality, while boys usually end up on the fourth stage with some expressions of the fifth and sixth stages of autonomous morality. Kohlberg is not surprised by this seeming deficiency in female moral development. He believes it is very functional for women who stay at home, where moral responsibility centers on helping and pleasing others. When these same women move into the traditional male areas of life they will, according to Kohlberg, come to "recognize the inadequacy of this moral perspective and progress like men toward higher stages where relationships are subordinated to rules (stage four) and rules to universal principles of justice (stages five and six)" (Gilligan, 1982, p. 18).

Piaget and Kohlberg both assume that males and females see moral problems in the same light, that of justice and personal rights, the highest form of moral development. Gilligan challenges this assumption with her studies of how young girls, college women, and housewives perceive the same moral problems Piaget and Kohlberg use. Women appear to frame moral problems in terms of conflicting personal responsibilities rather than as conflicting rights and abstract justice. "This conception of morality as concerned with the activity of care centers moral development around the understanding of responsibility and relationships, just as the conception of morality as fairness ties moral development to the understanding of rights and rules. This different construction of the moral problem by women may have been seen as the critical reason for their failure to develop within the constraints of Kohlberg's system" (Gilligan, 1982, p. 19).

Gilligan reminds us that the way people define moral problems, the situations they construe as moral conflicts in their lives, and the values they use in resolving them are all a function of their social conditioning. The boys Piaget studied loved to play highly structured games in which elaborate rules were necessary to resolve the inevitable conflicts. Adolescent boys focus first on developing their self-identity by separating themselves from others. Later on they develop their skill in intimacy and relationships.

The girls studied by Piaget and Gilligan, on the other hand, generally reacted differently. Their games were less structured and less competitive. They were more tolerant in their attitudes toward rules, more flexible in allowing exceptions, and more easily reconciled to innovations. When conflicts arose in their games, girls were more likely to stop the game to protect their relationships than to elaborate rules to resolve their disputes. Also, because of their subordinate role in society, the girls generally learned the meaning of their own identity and of intimacy simultaneously through their relationships.

From these differences Piaget and Kohlberg conclude that the legal sense, essential to moral development, is far less developed in little girls than in boys. Gilligan counters this assumption with this reminder:

The essence of moral decision is the exercise of choice and the willingness to accept responsibility for that choice. To the extent that women perceive themselves as having no choice (or power of self-determination), they correspondingly excuse themselves from the responsibility that decision entails. Childlike in the vulnerability of their dependence and consequent fear of abandonment, they claim to wish only to please, but in return for their goodness they expect to be loved and cared for. This is an "altruism" always at risk, for it presupposes an innocence constantly in danger of being compromised by an awareness of the trade-off that has been made. (Gilligan, 1982, p. 67)

Although Figure 2.1 illustrates the importance of social conditioning and social scripting for our moral decision making, it does not emphasize the importance of the very different social conditioning boys and girls receive. The world views (box A), desires and anxieties (box B), and objects, relations, and ideals (box C) are still very different for boys and girls in our American society.

Two Views of a Case Study

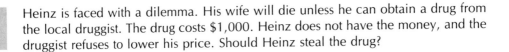

Heinz is faced with a dilemma. His wife will die unless he can obtain a drug from the local druggist. The drug costs $1,000. Heinz does not have the money, and the druggist refuses to lower his price. Should Heinz steal the drug?

FIGURE 2.1   *Social and environmental factors affecting our moral values. Whether we are a health care consumer or practitioner, we are subject to a variety of personal and environmental influences that condition and color the values we develop and the decisions we make. Below the broken horizontal line are the many personal factors we need to consider. Initially three elements, (A) our fixed or process world view (Chapter 1), (B) our emerging desires and concerns, and (C) our ideals, personal relationships, and experiences combine to create our personal values. These values are then given social expression in our laws, cultural values, and institutions. But science and technology also impact on our symbols and institutions, sometimes in a positive way, sometimes creating a disturbance or challenge (a cognitive dissonance). Filtered through our social institutions and symbols, our personal values are expressed in a particular lifestyle. The way we live as individuals then feeds back and impacts on our social and physical environment. The interaction between our personal lifestyles and the environment feeds back to us as individuals. As a result, we experience physical, biological, and social constraints. But the changing environment also impacts on our world view and leads to new desires or anxieties. Since this network of interacting factors is constantly changing for each one of us, we should be aware of these factors and how they might affect our decisions in biomedical ethics as well as other issues.*

(Reprinted from Howard Brody. *Ethical Decisions in Medicine.* Boston: Little, Brown, 1976, p. 288.)

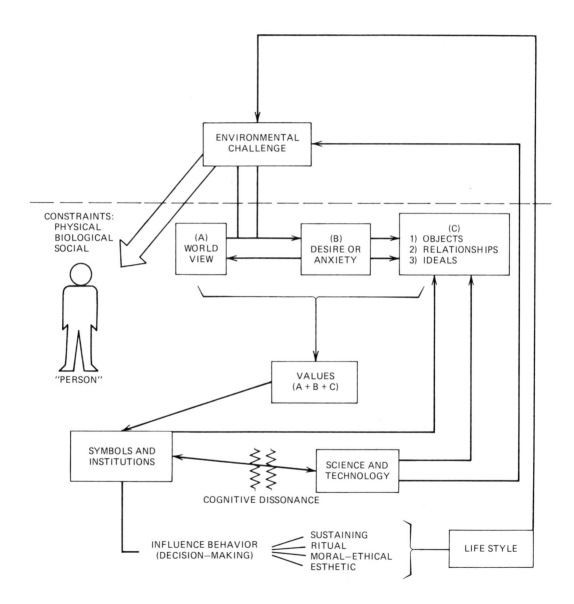

CONSTRAINTS:
PHYSICAL
BIOLOGICAL
SOCIAL

ENVIRONMENTAL
CHALLENGE

(A)
WORLD
VIEW

(B)
DESIRE OR
ANXIETY

(C)
1) OBJECTS
2) RELATIONSHIPS
3) IDEALS

"PERSON"

VALUES
(A + B + C)

SYMBOLS AND
INSTITUTIONS

SCIENCE AND
TECHNOLOGY

COGNITIVE DISSONANCE

INFLUENCE BEHAVIOR
(DECISION—MAKING)

SUSTAINING
RITUAL
MORAL—ETHICAL
ESTHETIC

LIFE STYLE

23

Asked to analyze this case, 11-year-old Jake came up with a very precise and logical solution:

A human life is worth more than money. Stealing the drug would not harm the druggist because he can recoup the loss by business with rich customers. Even if Heinz doesn't love his wife, he should steal the drug for her because if he is caught the judge will let him off lightly for "doing the right thing." (Gilligan, 1982, p. 26)

Jake's reasoning differentiates morality from law and admits that there may be some exceptions to laws against stealing. He is concerned about conflicts of abstract justice, between the right to private property and the right to live. This puts him on Kohlberg's level 5 or 6.

Amy, also 11, does not consider the issues of private property or law. She is concerned about the effect that Heinz's stealing would have on his relationship with his wife:

If he stole the drug, he might save his wife, but if he did, he might have to go to jail, and then his wife might get sicker again, and he couldn't get more of the drug, and it might not be good. So, they should really just talk it out and find some other way to get the money. (Gilligan, 1982, p. 28)

Amy is more concerned about the druggist's failure to respond to the need of Heinz and his wife than the violation of his private property. Amy's moral world is rooted in relationships and psychological truths, a belief in communications, the central ethic of care, and the responsibility of responding to another person's need. In Kohlberg's schema, Amy appears to have reached only level 3 or 4.

Female and Male Perspectives on Moral Problems

In summing up the main conclusions of her preliminary studies, Gilligan suggests four themes. First, there is a difference in initial moral imperative. For women, the initial moral imperative is an injunction to care for others, a responsibility to discern and alleviate the "real and recognizable trouble" of this world. For men, it is an injunction to respect the rights of others and in the process protect from infringement the rights to life and self-fulfillment.

Second, women's insistence on a caring ethic is at first self-critical rather than self-protective. Gradually, this absolute of caring becomes more complicated than its earliest definition of not hurting others because of a growing need for personal integrity. For men, their initial negative obligation of noninterference in the rights of others expands to recognizing the need for a more active responsibility in caring for others. For men, the absolutes of truth and fairness expand with experience into an ethic of generosity and care.

Third, as they move toward the postconventional morality on their own path, women come to see the personal violence that is contained in any inequality, whereas men come to see that their conception of justice cannot be blind to the differences in human life.

Finally, for both men and women, the existence of *two distinct contexts for moral decisions* makes our decisions relative to our gender and leads to a new understanding of responsibility and moral choice. However, the association of these two paths with gender—care with women and justice with men—is far from absolute. There appears, rather, to be an interplay of these two moral voices in both men and women with one or the other predominating in the beginning. Gradually the two voices converge and gain balance as a person matures in moral sensitivity.

Applying Models of Moral Development to Your Case Study

The models of moral development presented in this chapter have severe limitations. Piaget's and Kohlberg's models are conveniently structured and precise, but their male-biased assumptions and evidence are problems. Gilligan gives us preliminary insight into what may be a female path in moral thinking but without the convenience or detail of structured analysis. All three views need much more research before we can really claim to understand our development as moral persons. Meanwhile, we will attempt to apply and utilize their insights in an exercise to sharpen our sensitivity to the complexities of making moral decisions.

In the exercise in Part Two of this text you are asked to work out some ideas relevant to the two paths outlined in this chapter. The male path is fairly easy because it follows the six stages of Kohlberg's model, using the personal statements on the right side of Table 2.1. It focuses on justice and obvious personal rights. For this male side of the exercise you can also refer to Figure 1.2, which illustrates the logical, step-by-step methods of decision making, which appear more in the male path.

The female path is more difficult because you have only a brief summary of Gilligan's preliminary studies and a summary of Amy's comments to work with. If you are a woman, you can use this as a challenge to break away from the pressure to think logically in terms of justice and rights and to express your basic insights into a morality of care. If you are a man, you can accept a challenge to think creatively in a path you may not have used before.

Your instructor may assign you a brief case study to use as the basis for completing your exercise pages, or you may be allowed to select your own case study. In either event, make sure your case study has a central interpersonal relationship that will allow you to pursue both the male path of justice and rights and the female path of care and relationships.

REFERENCES AND FURTHER READINGS

Gilligan, C. *In a Different Voice.* Cambridge, MA: Harvard University Press, 1982.

Hersh, R. et al. *Promoting Moral Growth: From Piaget to Kohlberg.* New York: Longman, 1979.

Kohlberg, L. "Stage and sequence: The cognitive-developmental approach to socialization." In Goslin, D., ed. *Handbook of Socialization Theory and Research.* Chicago: Rand McNally, 1969.

Piaget, J. *The Moral Judgment of the Child.* New York: Free Press, 1965.

NOTES

Section II
Ethical Principles and Rules

3   IDENTIFYING ETHICAL PRINCIPLES

CHAPTER 3
IDENTIFYING
ETHICAL PRINCIPLES

In Chapter 1 we dealt with ethical systems, the most theoretical and general level of ethical reasoning. In Chapter 2 we explored the growing awareness of how our psychological development as males and females appears to condition our personal approach to ethical dilemmas. With this awareness of which ethical system is most in keeping with our convictions and a new sensitivity to our personal perspective, we can move to the second level of ethical thought, that of ethical principles.

Ethical principles are those general and fundamental truths, laws, or doctrines that we derive, often subconsciously, from our ethical system. Many people are well aware of their ethical principles but only vaguely aware that taken together as a whole these principles form an ethical system. At the same time, going in the other direction of our ethical hierarchy (Fig. 3.1), individual general principles are also used as the basis for the third level of ethical thinking, that of ethical rules. For example, the ethical principle that we must respect other persons is the basis for many specific ethical rules about telling the truth, not stealing, and not injuring others.

In Chapter 4 we explore the level of ethical rules. In the remaining chapters we concentrate on the most practical level of ethical thinking, that of judgments and decisions about how to act most ethically in a particular situation. In this hierarchy we are moving from the abstract and general to the concrete and particular.

As a starting point for our exploration of ethical principles, we can pose a specific problem: Is it ethical to involve children in research that is not therapeutic for them but that may ultimately benefit others? Assume that the research is scientifically and medically safe and acceptable. Assume that there is minimal or negligible risk to the child and that you have the legal consent of the child's parent or guardian. A classic example of this situation is the testing of the measles vaccine on mentally retarded children at Willowbrook on Staten Island, New York. This vaccine had been thoroughly tested on animals and proven both safe and effective, but until it was tested on humans, its actual effectiveness and safety could not be assured. The question is whether it was or was not

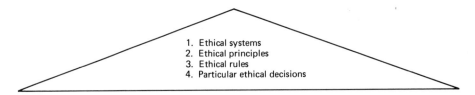

1. Ethical systems
2. Ethical principles
3. Ethical rules
4. Particular ethical decisions

FIGURE 3.1   *Four levels in the hierarchy of ethical thinking.*

ethical to test the vaccine on mentally retarded, institutionalized children, with consent of their parents.

The general principle we use in resolving this dilemma will vary, depending on which ethical system we follow.

When Paul Ramsey, a Kantian/biblical duty-oriented ethicist at Princeton Theological Seminary, approaches this problem, he uses the Kantian **principle of personal autonomy and respect for the human person.** In any situation we must ultimately maintain respect for personal independence and dignity, and never treat anyone as a means to some other end without their explicit consent. Ramsey sees medical research as a collaboration and coadventure, involving both the researcher and the subject. Grounded in Protestant biblical tradition of the covenant established by Christ among all people, he believes that this covenant requires full consent from both parties in any human relationship, including medical experimentation. Since the retarded child cannot consent to participate, Ramsey concludes that it is unethical to proceed with such research, regardless of the benefit to others and the lack of risk to the child. Ramsey sees participation in nontherapeutic research as a charitable act that the research subject must personally consent to (Ramsey, 1970, 1976).

When Richard McCormick, a natural-law, duty-oriented ethicist at the Kennedy Institute of Ethics at Georgetown University, approaches this same situation he applies a different principle. Instead of using the principle of personal autonomy, McCormick sees nontherapeutic research on minors as falling under the **principle of justice.** Under certain conditions he finds such research morally acceptable. These conditions include those mentioned above: research that is scientifically acceptable, poses minimal or no risk to the child, and is consented to by the child's parents or guardian. McCormick believes it is a matter of justice that we all ought to bear certain burdens and contribute, at least in some small way, to the common good. This is not only a charitable obligation but an obligation of justice we bear as members of the human race. McCormick argues that when the child *ought* to consent to nontherapeutic research out of its obligation of justice but cannot *give* consent, the child's legal guardian can and should consent in the child's place (McCormick, 1974, 1978).

Summary of Ethical Principles

Before we try to analyze and compare the ethical principles that form the basis for our professional codes of ethics, we need to complete our list of principles. While our focus here is that of the moral dimensions of health care, it should be mentioned that this list of principles obviously has equal implications and applications in other areas of human relations, such as politics, education, international relations, and business. As a starting point for our list we can use the outline by Beauchamp and Childress (1979).

Ramsey, as mentioned, uses one of the most important and basic ethical principles as the basis for his decision in the case of nontherapeutic research on minors, the **principle of autonomy.** Beauchamp and Childress (1979, p. 56) state that "autonomy is a form of personal liberty of action where the individual determines his or her own course of action in accordance with a plan chosen by himself or herself." Autonomy, in this definition, implies at least three elements: (1) the freedom to decide, (2) the freedom to act, and (3) acknowledgment and respect we owe the dignity and autonomy of others.

1. To decide freely, one needs to know all the facts available. Thus, a corollary of this principle of autonomy is that to make a free decision the person, first of all, "should have sufficient knowledge and comprehension of the subject matter involved as to enable him to make an understanding and enlightened decision" (The Nuremberg Code, rule 1).

2. However, one may have all the information one needs and still not be free to make one's own decision. Thus, a second corollary under the principle of autonomy requires that the person deciding "should be so situated as to be able to exercise free power of choice, without the intervention of any element of force, fraud, deceit, duress, over-reaching, or other ulterior form of constraint or coercion" (Nuremberg Code, rule 1).

Ethicists include these two subprinciples under the title of *informed consent.*

The freedom to act on one's own behalf, to implement one's free decision, might be stated in a paraphrase of the second subprinciple just cited from the Nuremberg Code. Thus, under the principle of personal autonomy everyone should be so situated as to be able to act on and implement their free choice, without the intervention of force, fraud, deceit, duress, over-reaching, or other ulterior form of constraint or coercion, within the limits of social good. The terminally ill cancer patient might freely decide to end all treatment or to take an overdose of medication to end his or her life. But if the family carefully monitors all medication, or if the patient is physically unable to carry out the decision, there is little effective personal autonomy.

These aspects of personal autonomy lead us to a variety of ethical rules governing the moral responsibility and rights of the health care professional and the patient. There are issues of the right to refuse treatment, the right to be thoroughly informed of all aspects of one's case, the right to refuse to participate in a procedure the health professional finds morally or professionally unacceptable, the right and/or responsibility of others to assist a helpless person in implementing his or her autonomous decision, and the right to end one's life.

3. Finally, we should mention that one can be autonomous and understand the autonomy of others in principle, but fail to apply this in a particular situation. Unfortunately, there is often a gap between recognizing the principle of autonomy and respecting it when one is personally involved in a health care relationship. If we expect others to respect our autonomy, then we need to grant the same respect for the autonomy of others, whatever the situation, within the requirements of the social good.

The principle of autonomy with its need for informed consent is linked with a second moral principle. The **principle of veracity** obligates both the health professional and the patient to tell the truth. Some ethicists question the absoluteness of this principle and argue that in the therapeutic setting there is such a thing as "benevolent deception." It may be more beneficial not to give the whole story or even deliberately to deceive the terminally ill patient or the person at high risk of developing an untreatable hereditary illness such as Huntington's disease, which brings premature brain deterioration and death. In addition, how do you respond to a patient who clearly indicates he or she does not want to know the whole story and prefers to leave decision making to you, based on your concern and expertise?

The third basic ethical principle, the **principle of nonmaleficence,** is clearly expressed in the Hippocratic oath which traditionally supports the medical profession: "I will never use treatment to injure or wrong the sick." In daily health care situations this principle has come to require the professional not to inflict any harm and to prevent evil or harm wherever possible.

Occasionally, the decision to do something for the good of the patient carries with it an inevitable secondary harmful effect. Performing an abortion may benefit the woman, but harms the fetus. Giving morphine to a terminally ill patient may relieve excruciating pain, but it may also directly hasten the patient's death. Some moralists resolve such dilemmas by applying the principle of double effect. They suggest that it is moral to act for the benefit of the patient and allow the second, harmful effect, provided the harm is not the means to the good end and provided the harm is not directly intended.

Some health professionals maintain that they must always do everything in their power to prolong the life of the patient. For example, these health professionals would believe that every effort must be made to save the life of a newborn with spina bifida because human life is of ultimate value. Others would interpret the principle of nonmaleficence in such situations to mean that it is often more humane and less harmful to allow nature to take its course without intervening with repeated major surgery to prolong the infant's life.

This principle raises the distinction of letting a patient die, indirectly "killing" the patient by not continuing treatment (passive euthanasia), and intervening to accelerate death (active euthanasia). It also raises the question of which treatments are morally obligatory and which are morally and medically optional, the difference between "ordinary" and "extraordinary" treatment. In making these distinctions, whose criteria do we use to decide what is obligatory/ordinary or optional/extraordinary?

Intimately associated with the principle of nonmaleficence is the **principle of beneficence.** Not only are health care providers ethically bound to respect the autonomy of patients and not to do them harm, they are also bound to contribute to their good health and welfare. In the words of the Hippocratic oath, a health professional pledges to "use treatment to help the sick according to my ability and judgment." Since everything we do both benefits and costs the patient, applying this principle opens the issue of analyzing the balance of benefits and costs, and determining whether the benefits truly outweigh the costs. The role of this issue in ethical decision making is the subject of exercises in Chapters 8, 9, and 11.

A fifth basic ethical principle of health care is the **principle of confidentiality.** Hippocrates touched on this moral principle when he wrote, "what I may see or hear in the course of the treatment or even outside of treatment of the patient in regard to the life of men, which on no account one must spread abroad, I will keep to myself, holding such things shameful to be spoken about." A modern version of the Hippocratic oath, the Declaration of Geneva, adopted by the General Assembly of the World Medical Association in 1948 (amended in 1968), is more terse: "I will respect the secrets which are confided in me, even after the patient has died."

This principle may sound simple and uncomplicated, but that is an illusion. The health professional is almost always dealing with more than the patient. In Chapter 6, when we examine the consequences of the implied social contract that exists between the patient and health professional, we will deal with some of the complications of confidentiality. For example, the rights and responsibilities of parents often conflict with rights of their sexually active teenage child to confidentiality when seeking a prescription contraceptive from a physician. This conflict arose in 1983 when the federal government ruled that federally funded clinics must notify in writing the parents of a minor who has received prescription contraceptives. Another example of this conflict occurs when a genetics counselor discovers a patient is a carrier of a crippling or lethal genetic disease and wishes to inform the patient's relatives of their risk but is bound to confidentiality by the patient. The patient's right to confidentiality often has to be balanced against the rights of others, including society.

Finally, there is the **principle of justice.** Beauchamp and Walters note that "the notion of justice has been analyzed in different ways in rival theories. But common to all theories of justice is this minimal principle: Like cases should be treated alike—or, to use the language of equality, equals ought to be treated equally and unequals unequally" (1982, p. 31). Under this principle, we encounter the issue of fair and equitable distribution of health care facilities and services, especially when there is not enough to meet everyone's needs. If, under the American Constitution, every person is "created equal," is an impartial lottery the most ethical way to distribute health services when we cannot afford to provide for everyone? Or, once the basic human rights "to life, liberty, and the pursuit of happiness" are met, should we consider each person's health care needs according to their individual effort, their merit, or their actual or potential contribution to society? What rules of justice should guide our priorities in allocating money and human resources in health care?

A list of the ethical principles follows:

1. Personal autonomy

2. Veracity

3. Nonmaleficence

4. Beneficence

5. Confidentiality

6. Justice

Phase One: Analyzing Ethical Principles in the Patient's Bill of Rights

Since the main focus of all health care delivery is the patient, it seems appropriate to start with a statement of what patients can rightfully expect of the health professionals serving their needs, from the staff physicians at a hospital or clinic to the nurses, technicians and therapists, social workers, and maintenance staff. All these people are part of the health care team. They are all, to some extent, both essential and responsible for the delivery of the best health care possible.

Though promoted by the American Hospital Association, the Patient's Bill of Rights below has no legal binding force. It does, however, contain guidelines derived from the six general ethical principles outlined above. Read the bill carefully and think about which ethical principle or principles are involved in each guideline or rule.

PATIENT'S BILL OF RIGHTS

The American Hospital Association presents a Patient's Bill of Rights with the expectation that observance of these rights will contribute to more effective patient care and greater satisfaction for the patient, his physician, and the hospital organization. Further, the Association presents these rights in the expectation that they will be supported by the hospital on behalf of its patients, as an integral part of the healing process. It is recognized that a personal relationship between the physician and the patient is essential for the provision of proper medical care. The traditional physician-patient relationship takes on a new dimension when care is rendered within an organizational structure. Legal precedent has established that the institution itself also has a responsibility to the patient. It is in recognition of these factors that these rights are affirmed.

	Autonomy	Veracity	Nonmaleficence	Beneficence	Confidentiality	Justice	Rank
1. The patient has the right to considerate and respectful care.							
2. The patient has the right to obtain from his physician complete current information concerning his diagnosis, treatment, and prognosis in terms the patient can be reasonably expected to understand. When it is not medically advisable to give such information to the patient, the information should be made available to an appropriate person in his behalf. He has the right to know by name the physician responsible for coordinating his care.							

3. The patient has the right to receive from his physician information necessary to give informed consent prior to the start of any procedure and/

Autonomy	Veracity	Nonmaleficence	Beneficence	Confidentiality	Justice	Rank

or treatment. Except in emergencies, such information for informed consent should include but not necessarily be limited to the specific procedure and/or treatment, the medically significant risks involved, and the probable duration of incapacitation. Where medically significant alternatives for care or treatment exist, or when the patient requests information concerning medical alternatives, the patient has the right to such information. The patient also has the right to know the name of the person responsible for the procedures and/or treatment.

4. The patient has the right to refuse treatment to the extent permitted by law, and to be informed of the medical consequences of his action.

5. The patient has the right to every consideration of his privacy concerning his own medical care program. Case discussion, consultation, examination, and treatment are confidential and should be conducted discreetly. Those not directly involved in his care must have the permission of the patient to be present.

6. The patient has the right to expect

Autonomy	Veracity	Nonmaleficence	Beneficence	Confidentiality	Justice	Rank

that all communications and records pertaining to his care should be treated as confidential.

7. The patient has the right to expect that within its capacity a hospital must make reasonable response to the request of a patient for services. The hospital must provide evaluation, service and/or referral as indicated by the urgency of the case. When medically permissible a patient may be transferred to another facility only after he has received complete information and explanation concerning the needs for and alternatives to such a transfer. The institution to which the patient is to be transferred must first have accepted the patient for transfer.

8. The patient has the right to obtain information as to any relationship of his hospital to other health care and educational institutions insofar as his care is concerned. The patient has the right to obtain information as to the existence of any professional relationships among individuals, by name, who are treating him.

9. The patient has the right to be advised if the hospital proposes to engage in or perform human experimentation affecting his care or

Autonomy	Veracity	Nonmaleficence	Beneficence	Confidentiality	Justice	Rank

treatment. The patient has the right to refuse to participate in such research projects.

10. The patient has the right to expect reasonable continuity of care. He has the right to know in advance what appointment times and physicians are available and where. The patient has the right to expect that the hospital will provide a mechanism whereby he is informed by his physician or a delegate of the physician of the patient's continuing health care requirements following discharge.

11. The patient has the right to examine and receive an explanation of his bill regardless of source of payment.

12. The patient has the right to know what hospital rules and regulations apply to his conduct as a patient.

No catalogue of rights can guarantee for the patient the kind of treatment he has a right to expect. A hospital has many functions to perform, including the prevention and treatment of disease, the education of both health professionals and patients, and the conduct of clinical research. All these activities must be conducted with an overriding concern for the patient, and, above all, the recognition of his dignity as a human being. Success in achieving this recognition assures success in the defense of the rights of the patient.

Now reread each of the 12 statements, keeping in mind the six principles outlined above. After each statement check in the appropriate box(es) the ethical principle(s) contained in that statement. Also, rank the ethical importance of each guideline on a scale of 5, for very important, to 1, minimally important.

Is any ethical principle not covered by the Patient's Bill of Rights? If so, how would you incorporate any missing principle in an amended version of this bill of rights?

_____

_____

_____

_____

_____

_____

_____

_____

_____

_____

_____

Phase Two: Analyzing Ethical Principles in the Ethical Code of the American Medical Association

The patient is one of two central persons in the health care situation. The physician, as head of the health care team, is the other. It is helpful to compare the ethical responsibilities of the physician as expressed in the 10-point ethical code of the American Medical Association with the Patient's Bill of Rights. Again, as you read each statement, check the appropriate box(es) after each guideline to indicate which of the six basic ethical principles is the source for that statement. Rank each statement for its ethical importance on a scale of 5, for very important, and 1, minimally important.

AMERICAN MEDICAL ASSOCIATION
PRINCIPLES OF MEDICAL ETHICS

Autonomy	Veracity	Nonmaleficence	Beneficence	Confidentiality	Justice	Rank

Preamble. These principles are intended to aid physicians individually and collectively in maintaining a high level of ethical conduct. They are not laws but standards by which a physician may determine the propriety of his conduct in his relationship with patients, with colleagues, with members of allied professions, and with the public.

Section 1. The principal objective of the medical profession is to render service to humanity with full respect for the dignity of man. Physicians should merit the confidence of patients entrusted to their care, rendering to each a full measure of service and devotion.

Section 2. Physicians should strive continually to improve medical knowledge and skill, and should make available to their patients and colleagues the benefits of their professional attainments.

Section 3. A physician should practice a method of healing founded on a scientific basis; and he should not voluntarily associate professionally with anyone who violates this principle.

Autonomy	Veracity	Nonmaleficence	Beneficence	Confidentiality	Justice	Rank

Section 4. The medical profession should safeguard the public and itself against physicians deficient in moral character or professional competence. Physicians should observe all laws, uphold the dignity and honor of the profession and accept its self-imposed disciplines. They should expose, without hesitation, illegal or unethical conduct of fellow members of the profession.

Section 5. A physician may choose whom he will serve. In an emergency, however, he should render service to the best of his ability. Having undertaken the care of a patient, he may not neglect him; and unless he has been discharged he may discontinue his services only after giving adequate notice. He should not solicit patients.

Section 6. A physician should not dispose of his services under terms or conditions which tend to interfere with or impair the free and complete exercise of his medical judgment and skill or tend to cause a deterioration of the quality of medical care.

Section 7. In the practice of medicine a physician should limit the source of his professional income to medical services actually rendered by him, or under his supervision, to his patients.

Autonomy	Veracity	Nonmaleficence	Beneficence	Confidentiality	Justice	Rank

His fee should be commensurate with the services rendered and the patient's ability to pay. He should neither pay nor receive a commission for referral of patients. Drugs, remedies or appliances may be dispensed or supplied by the physician provided it is in the best interests of the patient.

Section 8. A physician should seek consultation upon request; in doubtful or difficult cases; or whenever it appears that the quality of medical service may be enhanced thereby.

Section 9. A physician may not reveal the confidences entrusted to him in the course of medical attendance, or the deficiencies he may observe in the character of patients, unless he is required to do so by law or unless it becomes necessary to protect the welfare of the individual or of the community.

Section 10. The honored ideals of the medical profession imply that the responsibilities of the physician extend not only to the individual, but also to society where these responsibilities deserve his interest and participation in activities which have the purpose of improving both the health and the well-being of the individual and the community.

(Reprinted with permission of the American Medical Association.)

Are there any ethical principles not covered by this statement? If so, what additional rules or guidelines would you suggest?

_____

_____

_____

_____

_____

_____

_____

_____

_____

_____

_____

_____

_____

Analyzing Your Professional Code of Ethics

Having analyzed two professional codes of ethics, you can expand your knowledge and appreciation of ethical principles in the field of health care delivery by analyzing your own professional code or that of another allied health field. Several professional codes and parallel forms of analysis are given on pages 211–243 in Part Two of this worktext. You can choose from the Declaration of Geneva adopted by the World Medical Association, the International Code of Nursing Ethics, the Nuremberg Code on Permissible Medical Experiments, the International Code of Medical Ethics, the Declaration of Helsinki on Biomedical Research, the American Medical Association Ethical Guidelines for Clinical Investigation, the American Medical Technologists' Code of Ethics, the Code of Ethics of the American Society of Radiologic Technologists, the Code of Ethics for the American Physical Therapist Association, and the Code of Ethics for the American Association for Respiratory Therapy.

REFERENCES AND FURTHER READINGS

Beauchamp, T.L., & Childress, J.F. *Principles of Biomedical Ethics.* New York: Oxford University Press, 1979.

Fromer, M.J. *Ethical Issues in Health Care.* St. Louis: C.V. Mosby, 1981.

McCormick, R.A. "Proxy consent in the experimentation situation." *Perspectives in Biology and Medicine,* 1974, *18*(1), 2–20.

McCormick, R.A. "Proxy consent in the experimentation situation." In Beauchamp, T.L., & Walters, L. *Contemporary Issues in Bioethics.* Belmont, CA: Wadsworth, 1978.

Ramsey, P. *The Patient as Person.* New Haven: Yale University Press, 1970.

Ramsey, P. "Children in institutions." In Gorovitz, S. et al., eds. *Moral Problems in Medicine.* Englewood Cliffs, NJ: Prentice-Hall, 1976.

Ramsey, P. "The enforcement of morals: Nontherapeutic research on children." *Hastings Center Report.* 1976, *6*(4), 21–30.

Shelp, E.E., ed. *Beneficence and Health Care.* Hingham, MA: D. Reibel, 1982.

Shelp, E.E., ed. *Justice and Health Care.* Hingham, MA: D. Reibel, 1981.

Veatch, R.M. *A Theory of Medical Ethics.* New York: Basic Books, 1981.

NOTES

4 IDENTIFYING AND WEIGHTING ETHICAL RULES

CHAPTER 4
IDENTIFYING AND WEIGHTING ETHICAL RULES

In this chapter we identify and sort out the ethical rules or guidelines that can be derived from one of the ethical principles we identified in the previous chapter. This exercise helps us explore the third level of ethical thinking in the hierarchy of systems, principles, rules, and decisions. The principle selected for exploration here is the ethical principle of justice.

Some Distinctions in the Concept of Justice

Before we try to derive specific ethical rules and guidelines from the general principle, we need to make some distinctions and a brief outline of the way philosophers have subdivided the concept of justice.

The first distinction is between *retributive justice* and *distributive justice.* Since retributive justice deals with society's right to punish its members for behavior it considers criminal, it seldom arises in discussions of biomedical ethics. In recent years, however, one area of retributive justice has had considerable impact on our health care. This involves new and perplexing questions of *compensatory justice* (Purtillo & Cassel, 1981, pp. 192–200). How and to what extent is a private industry or government obligated to compensate the victims of industrial or environmental toxicity and job-related accidents? What compensation is owed and by whom to the people who live next to the thousands of toxic industrial waste dumps, such as the Love Canal neighborhood in Niagara, New York, or to the workers in asbestos plants and coal miners whose lung cancer is clearly linked to their workplace, or to pesticide workers who often become sterile because of their working environment?

Questions of distributive justice are very common in health care for two reasons. First, because we value health so highly in our culture, and second, because as a society we are always facing limitations in our ability to provide equal health care for our citizens. The fair and equitable division of health care resources is a major issue in distributive justice. We will deal with the practical problems of distributive justice in Chapter 5 when we try to select criteria that are fair and equitable in deciding who is to be treated in battle or in emergency situations, or when we face a shortage of equipment.

Our second distinction is between *formal justice* and *material justice*. Formal justice requires that "relevantly similar cases be treated in the same way and relevantly different cases in different ways" (McConnell, 1982, p. 198). The ethical concern in formal justice is that we apply the same criteria to all similar cases. Formal justice does not tell us whether or not our criteria are ethically valid or relevant. Can the requirements of formal justice easily support two patients being treated differently because one can pay and the other is on welfare? Under the principles of formal justice any criteria is acceptable, age, gender, size of family, race, religion, or need, provided that criterion is applied equally across the board.

Questions about what constitutes relevant or moral criteria shifts us into the domain of material justice. When advocates of competing theories of distributive or retributive justice disagree about what factors they should apply in determining punishment or a person's rights, they are dealing with material justice. In our exercise for this chapter we face the problem of identifying some criteria relevant to the principle of distributive justice in health care delivery.

Having established the difference between retributive, compensatory, and distributive justice, and between formal and material justice, we also need three other distinctions regarding the types of *rights* we derive from our principle of justice. As a preliminary, we should point out that there is a vital difference between a *right*, which is an obligation based on the principle of justice, and a *privilege*, which depends on the free will, kindness, or pleasure of another person. You have a right to your personal property that others have a moral obligation to respect. You do not thank others when they honor this moral obligation. On the other hand, when someone lends you a book, he or she is doing you a favor. Since you have no right or claim to the loan, an expression of gratitude is fully appropriate (McConnell, 1982, pp. 198–200).

Your right to something can be either a *moral right*, a *legal right*, or a right based on *both moral and legal obligations*.

Your right to something may also be *natural*—owed to you in virtue of your human nature. Or your right can be *voluntarily incurred*—based on a contract or relationship you and someone else freely enter into.

Our third distinction is between rights that are *in rem* and *in personam. In rem* rights obligate everyone and the whole society. They are usually stated in the negative. The right to "no taxation without representation," and the right not to be murdered or tortured are examples of *in rem* rights. Whether positive *in rem* rights exist, such as the right of every citizen to adequate health care or the right of an accident victim to be helped by any passer-by, is hotly debated by ethicists.

In personam rights obligate only some individuals in a society because these individuals have entered into a voluntary contractual agreement. The implied social contract between the patient and the individual health care professional, which we will examine in Chapter 6, contains typical *in personam* rights and responsibilities.

In summary, we have

1. Retributive justice including compensatory justice versus distributive justice

2. Formal justice versus material justice

3. Morally, legally, or both morally and legally based rights

4. Natural or contractual rights

5. *In rem* and *in personam* rights

Finally, we need to be aware that in the area of distributive justice there is a wide range of theories and positions. However vague and imprecise the common labels of "conservative" or "right wing" and "liberal" or "left wing" are, they do represent two ends of a spectrum of views on what constitutes a just society. Such a society's members are concerned about the fair and just distribution of economic goods. These economic goods pertain to our survival, that is, our needs for shelter, food, clothing, jobs, and equitable wages. But the economic goods can also include benefits such as leisure time, retirement benefits, and health care, including the possibility of national health insurance or socialized medicine (McConnell, 1982, pp. 201–229).

Despite the variety and range of views, those who take a conservative approach to distributive justice are generally inclined to emphasize personal property rights and individual freedom. Charity might encourage individuals to contribute to the health care of the indigent and poor, but there is no obligation in justice that would allow taxing the rich to provide for the poor. Those who take a liberal view of distributive justice argue that we are morally obligated to create a society with as little social and economic inequality as possible. In this view every citizen has a positive *in rem* right to adequate health care and a basic standard of living.

The implications of this conservative–liberal spectrum, along with the contrasting world views and male–female perspectives examined in Chapters 1 and 2, are applied to health care in phase 1 of our sample exercise below.

Phase One

Before you attempt to deduce the various health-related guidelines inherent in the principle of distributive justice, you should identify your own personal conservative–liberal bias and link this with the contrasting world views and the male–female gender bias we examined in Chapters 1 and 2. In this exercise, as in any ethical discussion, it is important to be aware of these personal orientations and the ways in which they will color and affect all the rules you draw from the general principle of distributive justice.

Below are six statements related to distributive justice controversies in health care. Each statement has a continuum or spectrum beneath it. Indicate your agreement or disagreement by circling your position in the spectrum of views below each statement.

Statement 1: The less distance that exists between the "better off" and the "worse off" in a society, the more distributive justice is valued and effectively practiced by the citizens.

Agree strongly	Agree	Not certain	Disagree	Disagree strongly

Statement 2: People are not morally bound to structure the economies of their society so that the well-off are taxed to support or improve the lot of less fortunate people.

Agree strongly	Agree	Not certain	Disagree	Disagree strongly

Statement 3: Government should not regulate the free enterprise system and private businesses.

Agree strongly	Agree	Not certain	Disagree	Disagree strongly

Statement 4: Because they are part of our free enterprise system, physicians and health care professionals should be free to engage in work slow-downs and selective strikes in order to force an equitable salary scale or rectify harmful work conditions when other means fail.

Agree strongly	Agree	Not certain	Disagree	Disagree strongly

Statement 5: The benefits of a national health care and insurance program clearly outweigh the loss of individual autonomy and the weakened financial situation of medical workers.

Agree strongly	Agree	Not certain	Disagree	Disagree strongly

Statement 6: A national health insurance system should be adopted by Congress and funded on a federal level to make sure every American receives at least a minimum level of health care.

Agree strongly	Agree	Not certain	Disagree	Disagree strongly

To learn your conservative/liberal bias on these issues, check your circled answers for each statement and total up your points as follows:

Statements 1, 5, and 6: Agree strongly = 1 point; Agree = 2 points; Not certain = 3 points; Disagree = 4 points; and Disagree strongly = 5 points.

Statements 2, 3, and 4: Agree strongly = 5 points; Agree = 4 points; Not certain = 3 points; Disagree = 2 points; and Disagree strongly = 1 point.

A total of six points is very much on the liberal side of the spectrum, whereas a score of 30 represents a very conservative approach to distributive justice issues in health care. Keep in mind that you may be quite liberal or conservative on one issue, and the exact opposite on another issue.

How does your position on the conservative–liberal spectrum relate to your orientation in terms of fixed versus process world views? Can you discern any relationship between your views on these two spectra, and your gender-based outlook on rights and responsibilities versus the impact on relationships?

Phase Two

In this section is a list of topics or issues related to distributive and compensatory justice in society and the health care system. Your task is to use these topics and issues as a springboard to create a list of rules or practical guidelines in keeping with your basic conservative or liberal bias. This list can be shared in class discussion.

ISSUES AND TOPICS RELATED TO JUSTICE IN THE HEALTH CARE SYSTEMS

- The individual's right to basic health care and society's obligation to provide it.

- Regulation of the distribution of health care professionals to provide for areas with insufficient numbers of skilled personnel.

- Regulation of skyrocketing health care costs.

- Distribution of monies to support basic research, technological advances, preventive medicine programs, and esoteric and very expensive treatments.
- Establishment of priorities to reduce inequalities in the availability of health care services.
- The right of health professionals to unionize, engage in slow-downs, and strike.
- Guidelines to direct the allocation of scarce resources or equipment.
- The use of merit, individual need, individual effort, and/or societal contribution as criteria for distributive justice.
- Health care rights in situations of self-created health problems (e.g., lung cancer and emphysema in the heavy smoker, hepatitis in the drug addict, liver and kidney problems in the alcoholic, and obesity in the cardiac patient).
- The use of certain classes of people—prisoners, minors, the mentally retarded and institutionalized—for experimentation and the testing of drugs.
- Regulation or limitation by tax disincentives or other means of the right of persons to reproduce when they are known to be at risk for passing on serious crippling inherited diseases to their offspring.
- Differential health insurance rates for smokers and heavy drinkers.
- Funding priorities for crisis interventions such as kidney dialysis, artificial heart implants, and heart transplants for a small number of persons in contrast to less politically popular preventive medicine programs for large numbers of people.
- Criteria for selection of individuals to receive scarce treatment such as a kidney transplant or dialysis.
- The responsibility of employers and industries to provide a healthy and safe environment for their workers.
- The definition of "just" health care delivery.
- The right of workers to know the health risks of their employment and the right to refuse health hazards in the workplace.
- The responsibility for and the types of professional peer reviews.
- Compensation to the victims of industrial pollution.
- Denouncing incompetent or unethical colleagues.
- Solidarity among health care colleagues.

- Government regulation of continuing professional education, licensing, and updating.

- Decisions of who lives and who dies when there are not enough resources to save all and what criteria are used.

- The "contract" between patient and health care professional.

Your statements of rules and guidelines can be phrased in several ways:

"Society should . . ."

". . . have a right to . . ."

"Health professionals are responsible for (or should) . . ."

"Distribution of . . . ought to be based on . . ."

". . . are responsible for . . ."

". . . should be required to . . ."

". . . should never . . ."

". . . ought to . . ."

The use of such terms as *ought, should,* and *has a right to* indicates a moral obligation. This is because in this exercise we are interested in deriving moral rules from the ethical principle of justice and weighting these in terms of their importance. Share and discuss your lists in class. Your instructor may also ask you to polish your list and hand it in.

YOUR LIST OF RULES AND GUIDELINES

_____

_____

_____

_____

_____

_____

_____

_____

Phase Three

Using your list of justice-oriented rules, select 10 statements at random or pick 10 guidelines that you believe are more important. Your next task is to arrange these 10 statements in a hierarchy indicating their importance to you. Pick a couple of key words in each statement to identify it and then arrange your 10 rules in the space provided in Table 4.1. Put your most important moral guideline at the top of the list and the least important statement at the bottom. If two or more values are equally important to you and carry about the same moral weight, list these one after the other. We will indicate the equality of such statements in our next step (see Statements numbered 2, 5, 6, 8, and 10 in Table 4.2).

TABLE 4.1   Hierarchy of Rules

Statement of Rule[a]	Order Number	Weighting Factor
1.		
2.		
3.		
4.		
5.		
6.		
7.		
8.		
9.		
10.		
TOTAL =		

[a]Identify rule by key words.

Having ranked your 10 rules, you can now indicate their relative importance and relation to each other by giving each rule an order number. In Table 4.2, by giving the most important rule a 10 and the next statement a 7, we indicate that we see the first statement as a much more serious moral obligation than the second statement. Giving Statements 2, 5, and 10 the same order number of 6 puts them on a par. The gap between the ordering of the first and second statements is larger than the gap we see at the bottom of the hierarchy, indicating another subtlety in the hierarchy of priorities.

The next step is to calculate the weighting factor for each of your moral statements.* To do this add up the order numbers. In our example, the total is 49. To determine the weighting factor for the first statement in Table 4.2 we divide the order number we gave it, 10, by our total, 49. The weighting factor (WF) for the first statement is $10 \div 49 = 0.204$. For the second statement, we have $7 \div 49 = 0.142$. This division procedure is repeated for all the other statements.

No matter how you arrange your moral statements in this hierarchy, you need only add up the order numbers you assigned and divide this total into the order number for each statement to obtain its weighting factor.

The weighting factors are a common way of giving a quantitative measure to different items in a list. Your first list of rules in Table 4.1 was a very rough sorting of priorities. Assigning an order number added a little more precision, which was then refined by the weighting factors.

TABLE 4.2 Example of the Ranking and Weighting of 10 Statements

Moral Value	Order	Weighting Factor
Statement 7	10	$10 \div 49 = 0.204$
Statement 4	7	$7 \div 49 = 0.142$
Statement 2	6	$6 \div 49 = 0.122$
Statement 10	6	$6 \div 49 = 0.122$
Statement 5	6	$6 \div 49 = 0.122$
Statement 9	5	$5 \div 49 = 0.102$
Statement 7	4	$4 \div 49 = 0.081$
Statement 3	3	$3 \div 49 = 0.061$
Statement 6	1	$1 \div 49 = 0.020$
Statement 8	1	$1 \div 49 = 0.020$
TOTAL 49		$49 \div 49 = 1.000$

*From here on, a pocket calculator will be very handy.

Using This Technique to Identify and Weight Rules

In the exercise on pages 245–251 in Part Two of this text you will be asked (1) to identify your position on the conservative-liberal spectrum, (2) to create a list of rules related to the principle of personal autonomy, and (3) to refine your priorities using the order number and weighting factor technique of decision making.

REFERENCES AND FURTHER READINGS

Barry, V. *Moral Aspects of Health Care.* Belmont, CA: Wadsworth, 1982, pp. 17–48, 467–499.

Beauchamp, T.L., & Walters, L., eds. *Contemporary Issues in Bioethics,* 2nd ed. Belmont, CA: Wadsworth, 1982, pp. 381–502.

Fromer, M.J. *Ethical Issues in Health Care.* St. Louis: C.V. Mosby, 1981, pp. 35–65.

Kieffer, G.H. *Bioethics: A Textbook of Issues.* Reading, MA: Addison-Wesley, 1979, pp. 379–412.

McConnell, T.C. *Moral Issues in Health Care.* Monterey, CA: Wadsworth Health Sciences, 1982, pp. 197–232.

Purtillo, R.B., & Cassel, C.K. *Ethical Dimensions in the Health Professions.* Philadelphia: W.B. Saunders, 1981, pp. 181–208.

Shannon, T.A., ed. *Bioethics: Basic Writings.* New York: Paulist Press, 1981, pp. 477–555.

Shelp, E.E., ed. *Justice and Health Care.* Hingham, MA: D. Reibel, 1981.

Section III
Techniques for Making Ethical Decisions

5 DECISIONS IN TRIAGE SITUATIONS

CHAPTER 5
DECISIONS IN TRIAGE SITUATIONS

One of the most perplexing and disturbing problems of medical ethics is that of making decisions about who should receive medical treatment when only a few of those needing treatment can be accommodated.

Such a problem arose during the 1943 American campaign against Rommel's Nazi army in North Africa. The prime objective of the military was to defeat Rommel's forces quickly with as few casualties as possible. Penicillin had just been discovered and was in very short supply. The lives of many seriously wounded soldiers could be saved with the new antibiotic, returning them to battle. However, many more soldiers were incapacitated by venereal diseases contracted from prostitutes and native women. With penicillin these men could be returned to battle more quickly.

Since there was not enough penicillin to treat both groups, the decision rested on what Paul Ramsey calls "focused criteria." The drug was given to the soldiers with VD, although this meant that many of those wounded in battle would die. The prime criterion or ethical objective for the decision was to have as many functional soldiers as possible in order to win the battle quickly while keeping the total loss of human life as low as possible.

In the television series M*A*S*H, based on the experiences of mobile army surgical hospitals during the Korean War, the medical team of Hawkeye Pierce, Charles Emerson Winchester, B.J. Honeycut, Margaret Houlihan, her nurses, and Colonel Henry Blake drops everything when Radar's voice comes over the public address system with the call of "TRIAGE, TRIAGE—Helicopters with wounded now arriving!" The 1960 Webster's dictionary did not include *triage* and few people outside the medical setting knew its meaning. However, as a result of the Vietnam War and of television cameras filming the medical teams at the sites of major disasters, our understanding has changed. In November 1979, a fire at the MGM Hotel in Las Vegas killed 84 persons. On October 23, 1980, a powerful explosion ripped through an elementary school in Ortuella, Spain, just before noon, killing 64 persons, mostly children, and injuring more than 100. On December 4, 1980, a fireball swept through the conference rooms of the Stouffer Inn at Harrison, New York; 26 people were killed and over 40 were seriously injured. On July 17, 1981, the posh jammed ballroom of the

Kansas City Hyatt-Regency Hotel became mayhem when two walkways collapsed; 111 people died and over 190 were injured. Today when such tragedies occur, television cameras are on the spot reporting the realities of triage. But medical personnel face many less sensational examples of triage every day.

The *American Heritage Dictionary* now gives two definitions for *triage*. First, triage is defined as "a system designed to produce the greatest benefit from limited treatment facilities for battlefield casualties by giving treatment to those who may survive with proper treatment and not to those who have no chance of survival and those who will survive without it." In the second definition, triage is "any system used to allocate a scarce commodity, such as food, only to those capable of deriving the greatest benefit from it."

Triage in Modern Medicine

The 1943 decision of the medical commander in the African theater to give penicillin to men "wounded in brothels" instead of to those wounded in battle was justified by the special criterion of national survival during war. In that situation ethical primacy was given to the utilitarian objective of the greatest social good for the most people, even though this violates the duty-oriented interpretation of justice.

Warfare is the classic setting for triage. The wounded are divided into three groups. The "walking wounded" whose superficial wounds require only minimal care are ignored and not treated in the emergency situation. Some individuals in this group might be selected for treatment to return them to usefulness as soon as possible. A physician or nurse with superficial injuries, for instance, might be treated to increase her or his efficiency in helping others. The second group, those fatally injured, might be given pain killers but would be allowed to die since no amount of treatment could save them. The third group includes the seriously wounded, where the concentration of medical attention will result in the largest percentage of survivors.

These same three groups can be found at the site of any disaster. The emergency mobile units, paramedics, physicians, and others who arrive first at the hotel fires, school explosion, and building collapse mentioned above reacted professionally, making rapid decisions about who to treat first. Almost instinctively the injured were divided into the three groups mentioned. Despite their pain, some could wait for treatment without danger of dying. Others were injured beyond hope of recovery. In the stress of a crisis when available skilled personnel and equipment are limited, treating as many of the seriously injured as you can in hope of saving as many as possible becomes an ethical priority.

Though in theory every single person at a disaster site has an equal right to life-saving treatment, triage is the reality. Treatment cannot be available on a "first come, first served" basis, nor can a random lottery or factors such as race, age, social position, or apparent wealth be used to decide who is treated under these special circumstances.

When patients from the first on-site selection arrive at the emergency rooms of nearby hospitals, another triage selection process may begin. In the stress of a dozen ambulances arriving almost simultaneously at the emergency room, physicians may rely on the judgment of other health professionals trained in emergency procedures to evaluate triage prospects. Still later, in a much calmer setting, triage decisions may again be needed in the intensive care unit of the hospital.

Triage is commonly justified and practiced in the crisis of war or disaster. But is it equally ethical in other situations? For instance, how should the candidates for kidney dialysis be selected when the need exceeds the equipment and skilled personnel available? Should selection be based on a first come, first treated basis? Or is a lottery a more just way to allocate scarce medical care? Dialysis today is a common treatment that the federal government has decided should come under our health insurance, but it had once been considered experimental and extraordinary. If everyone has an equal right to life, does everyone also have an equal right to experimental and extraordinary care? Or is the right to treatment limited to equitable distribution and access to basic health care?

If the right to be treated must be limited, then what criteria should we use? In terms of material justice, which we first explored in Chapter 3, our criteria might be

1. Everyone has the same equal right, decided by lottery or first come, first treated.

2. Every person should be treated in proportion to his or her need.

3. Everyone should be treated according to his or her previous effort or work.

4. People should be selected for treatment on the basis of their actual or potential contribution to society.

5. People should be selected for treatment depending on their merit.

6. Treatment should be based on the ability to pay.

As Beauchamp and Childress point out (1979, p. 173), most societies use all six of these criteria for selection in the allocation of scarce resources, depending on the circumstances. Unemployment benefits are given on the basis of previous effort, one's length of employment. Aid to dependent children and welfare support are given on the basis of need. Jobs and promotions are distributed on the basis of merit and effort. The higher salaries and fees of some professionals are justified in terms of their effort (time spent in training), their special skills, or their contribution to society.

Those who follow consequence-oriented ethics may be more inclined to suggest criteria other than a lottery or queuing up as a solution to the issues of equitable distribution of scarce resources and treatment. Duty-oriented ethicists are more likely to hold for the lottery or first come first served criteria.

A BRIEF ILLUSTRATION

If your intensive care unit had only one extracorporeal membrane oxygenator (ECMO)—an artificial lung—how would you handle the following situation? The patient now on the ECMO is 86 years old. A new patient, age 36, with multisystem failure and severe trauma needs the ECMO to live. You cannot get a second ECMO, and neither patient can be transferred. How would you judge their "relative merits"? Would you consider taking the 86-year-old off the artificial lung so the 36-year-old can live? What would you do if the older patient were an addict from skid row and the younger patient the mother of five young children? Would your decision be more difficult or easier if the younger patient were the father and sole supporter of five young children or were an unmarried teenager? Would your decision be affected if one of the patients could not pay for the treatment? What would you do if the second patient had previously donated the money to purchase the ECMO and establish a scholarship to train the specialist needed to run the machine? Without the effort and generosity of this one person the hospital would not have had the ECMO or personnel to save dozens of lives.

Questions of criteria are central to making triage decisions, as we will see in the rest of this chapter and in our exercise. Applying the above six criteria to our two patients needing the ECMO brings some important insights.

Under the first criterion (p. 65), both patients have an equal right to the ECMO. If both had arrived at the same time, a lottery would have been appropriate. But since the older person arrived first and is already on the ECMO, the other person is out of luck despite merit, need, and so forth. Under the second criterion, relative need, both patients are equally in need of life-saving equipment. We might therefore revert back to our first criterion.

Our third criterion, one's effort, raises a new issue. Does the fact that the second patient donated the ECMO and paid for training the staff give that patient a priority, even if it means removing the first patient from the life-saving treatment? What if the older patient really has very little will to live but won't make the decision to refuse further treatment, whereas the younger patient has a very strong will to recover which makes her prospects for recovery far better? What if the older patient needs the ECMO because of life-threatening injuries incurred in an accident while driving under the influence of alcohol, whereas the second patient is the innocent victim of a drunk driver? Are these facts relevant or irrelevant in our ethical decision?

The fourth criterion brings into play several factors that are difficult, if not impossible, to quantify. How do you determine and compare the actual or potential societal value of two human beings? Are such factors as marital or parental status important to an ethical decision? Is social status a valid factor? Does it matter that one is a president, a "hippy," or an addict? Is one's gender or age important? Should women and children really come first? The same questions are relevant when we try to use merit as a factor to resolve the distribution of a limited amount of life-saving equipment when the need exceeds the availability.

CASE STUDY: TRIAGE IN A LIFEBOAT

In 1842 a sailing ship sank after striking an iceberg in the north Atlantic. The crew and half of the passengers escaped in two lifeboats. One was so overcrowded it began to leak and flounder in the high seas. The desperate crew decided on a triage ethic in which all the women and married men would be saved. Fourteen single men were thrown overboard and two of their sisters voluntarily jumped over with them. A few hours later the remaining survivors were rescued. Back in Philadelphia, the crew quickly disappeared, leaving only one crewman, Seaman Holmes, to be tried in court.

The defense argued along consequential lines that since it was unlikely that anyone would volunteer to jump overboard to save the others, the sailors had chosen the most ethical solution. The defense argument was that the most ethical way to resolve the right to a life-saving seat in the floundering lifeboat was to decide on a combination of consequences and duties. In Victorian times, keeping marriages and families intact was an important consequence. Protecting "defenseless" women and children was an important duty. In a crisis single men should be the first to go.

The judge, however, followed a different duty-oriented approach to justice and used the first of our six criteria above. A lottery was the only ethical solution since every person in the lifeboat had an equal right to life. Seaman Holmes was convicted of homicide. Thus the concept of "lifeboat ethics" was born.

Over a century later, Garrett Hardin, a leader in the movement to control overpopulation, applied this lifeboat ethic to planet Earth. Instead of sailors and passengers fighting for the right to survive, the nations of the earth and their citizens are constantly fighting and bickering for their own advantage.

Each rich nation amounts to a lifeboat full of comparatively rich people. The poor of the world are in other, much more crowded lifeboats. Continuously, so to speak, the poor fall out of their lifeboats and swim for a while in the water hoping to be admitted to a rich lifeboat, or in some other way to benefit from the "goodies" on board. (Hardin, 1974)

The United States is very attractive as a "lifeboat." In 1979 and 1980, over 110,000 Cuban refugees fled to the shores of Florida. Thousands of Haitians fled economic and political repression in their Carribean homeland. The Vietnamese and Cambodian "boat people" came by the thousands. Each year over three million Mexicans cross the border into the southwestern United States. It is predicted that by 1990, two-thirds of all Californians will be recent immigrants from "sinking lifeboats" in the South Pacific, Latin America, and the Far East. By 1990, experts predict, one in four residents of the United States will belong to what we now call "minorities." How realistic, then, is Hardin's application of triage criteria to our immigration and foreign aid policies?

Daniel Callahan has asked some crucial questions about the use of "lifeboat ethics" and triage as a solution to the problems of world population and immigration which clearly illustrate the complexities of triage and the difficulty in making truly ethical decisions (Callahan, 1974).

First, Callahan questions the assumption that some nations can stay afloat even while other nations flounder on the verge of disaster and starvation. Hardin's lifeboats appear independent of each other and thus their fates seem to be independent. That may have been a valid image of the nations of the world in the past, but today the interdependence of nations is a painful reality. The Falkland Islands dispute between Great Britain and Argentina, the wars in the Near East between Arab nations and Israel or between Iran and Iraq, tensions between Nationalist China and the Peoples Republic of China, and countless other political conflicts link our "lifeboats" with unbreakable chains of interdependence.

Most of the basic industrial raw materials that keep the United States affluent come from other nations. One hundred percent of our chromium, manganese, and tin come from the developing nations. By 1985, over 90% of our needs for aluminum and over 80% of our needs for nickel and tungsten will be met by the "sinking lifeboats." In simple terms 6% of the people in the lifeboats are consuming about 40% of the world's resources.

As a second point against applying triage to our overpopulated world, Callahan argues that the nations of Europe and North America are to some extent responsible for the plight of other nations. By getting a head start on other nations in terms of economic and industrial development, the developed nations have been able to accelerate their own growth by exploiting the underdeveloped nations for cheap resources. You may recall that a decade ago we paid $2 or $3 a barrel for oil from the Near East and 20 cents a gallon for gasoline to run our cars. In 1982 we paid over $30 a barrel and well over $1 per gallon at the pump because of the new-found economic power of the countries in the Persian Gulf and Latin America.

Margot Fromer adds another insight when she comments that "discrimination between classes of people is morally justified only if properties of the groups are the moral responsibility of the group members or if they are the sort of properties that can be overcome" (1981, p. 40). The poverty, mass starvation, and overpopulation of many nations today is not something for which the individuals in these countries are responsible. Cultural, economic, religious, political, and other circumstances have given European and North American nations the edge in survival and greatly reduced the ability of the poor nations to repair their "leaky boat" without help from the more advantaged.

As his third point, Callahan asks what we might do to expand the carrying capacity of the "leaky boats." The development of agricultural resources with new hybrids and more efficient farming, equitable payment for raw resources, the application of appropriate soft technologies and the encouragement of population control are remedies that the developed nations can provide to stabilize the unbalanced world without revolution and violence.

Hardin views Callahan's criticisms as idealistic and impractical. Generosity on the part of the rich nations, trying to share their wealth and lifestyle, will only hasten the day of disaster for all. He believes it is impossible for all to survive and also impossible to find an ethical basis on which to select survivors. Joseph Fletcher, author of *Situation Ethics,* agrees, pointing out that the charity of rich nations sending high protein food to the poor nations is not moral because it only worsens their situation. High protein food increases the fertility rate of the poor and results in more people to starve in future years.

A practical application of this debate will be used in Phase Two of the exercise for this chapter.

Origins of Triage Decisions

Outside of unexpected disasters and the unavoidable shortages that plague warfare, the triage ethics we face in health care—the shortages of equipment and skilled professionals and food to feed starving populations—are inevitably rooted in our past decisions about priorities. As individuals and as nations, our decisions about where and in what proportions we want to invest our time, energy, and money have created and continue to exacerbate the problems of limited equipment and other shortages we face.

As an illustration, we might cite the present concern over genetic diseases in the United States. About 44,000 Americans suffer from Down's syndrome, which results from an extra twenty-first chromosome. Two hundred thousand people suffer from inherited muscular dystrophy, 248,000 from congenital heart defects, 10,000 from cystic fibrosis, 16,000 from sickle cell anemia, and over 12,000 from hemophilia. One in every 16 infants born in the United States and Canada suffers from one or more congenital malformations so severe that it will die or be severely handicapped for life unless treated. It has been estimated that it would take 50,000 man-years of research effort and $5 billion to give us a detailed understanding of the hereditary information contained in the genes on our 46 human chromosomes.

In view of our current primitive knowledge of human genetics and our startling advances in other areas such as space technology, it is apparent that human genetic research has not been given a high priority. In fact, the nations of the world have invested all the manpower and money we would need to understand fully the human genetic code in their military budget for just three days of 1981! As a consequence, we face triage situations in genetic screening programs and in our war on congenital and hereditary diseases.

On the worldwide level, the developed nations devote less than 1% of their gross national product to aid for the developing nations. This 0.7% compares with 6% of the world's gross national product that is devoted to the military. Each year, the developed nations provide over 25 times more military aid than they do other assistance to the underdeveloped nations. A shift in our priorities of only 10% of the world's expenditure on the military to other assistance could increase the nonmilitary aid to underdeveloped nations by 33%.

Our decisions about priorities, then, have contributed to our triage decisions at home and abroad. Our priorities and decisions on the proportion of our national budget that we want to devote to social programs, medical research, and armament set the stage for limited equipment in local health care. They also color our discussion and current decisions in dealing with the crisis of overpopulation in the underdeveloped nations and our moral responsibilities in that regard.

Applying Triage Criteria to Your Case Studies

The points raised in this chapter regarding triage decisions are far from comprehensive. However, I have tried to pick out some of the main issues and arguments that you can use in two brief triage exercises. The first case study given in the exercise in Part Two deals with a shortage of life-sustaining equipment. The second case study deals with triage on an international scale.

These two exercises are not as structured as other exercises in this worktext. Therefore, you have freedom to think on your own. You may prefer the more structured questions of other exercises, but being forced to integrate the general ideas presented in this chapter with your own thinking about the issues and questions is necessary to gain a broader sensitivity and skill in making decisions.

REFERENCES AND FURTHER READINGS

Barry, V. *Moral Aspects of Health Care.* Belmont, CA: Wadsworth, 1982, pp. 17–48, 467–499.

Beauchamp, T.L., & Childress, J.F. *Principles of Biomedical Ethics.* New York: Oxford University Press, 1979.

Beauchamp, T.L., & Walters, L., eds. *Contemporary Issues in Bioethics,* 2nd ed. Belmont, CA: Wadsworth, 1982, pp. 381–502.

Callahan, D. "Doing well by doing good." *Hastings Center Report,* 1974, 4(6), 1–4.

Fletcher, J. *Situation Ethics: The New Morality.* Philadelphia: Westminster Press, 1966.

Fromer, M.J. *Ethical Issues in Health Care.* St. Louis: C.V. Mosby, 1981, pp. 35–65.

Hardin, G. "Living on a lifeboat." *Bioscience,* 1974, 24(10), 561–568.

Kieffer, G.H. *Bioethics: A Textbook of Issues.* Reading, MA: Addison-Wesley, 1979, pp. 379–412.

McConnell, T.C. *Moral Issues in Health Care.* Monterey, CA: Wadsworth Health Sciences, 1982, pp. 197–232.

Purtillo, R.B., & Cassel, C.K. *Ethical Dimensions in the Health Professions.* Philadelphia: W.B. Saunders, 1981, pp. 181–208.

Shannon, T.A., ed. *Bioethics: Basic Writings.* New York: Paulist Press, 1981, pp. 477–555.

Shelp, E.E., ed. *Justice and Health Care.* Hingham, MA: D. Reibel, 1981.

Schwartz, H. "Rationing medicine." *The New York Times,* July 30, 1982, p. A25.

6 THE SOCIAL CONTRACT BETWEEN PATIENT AND HEALTH CARE WORKER

CHAPTER 6
THE SOCIAL CONTRACT
BETWEEN PATIENT
AND HEALTH CARE WORKER

In every health care situation, there are two central persons, one in need of skilled sensitive care and the other seeking to fill that need. The personal network, however, includes also the patient's family and the members of the health care team besides the physician. Of all the elements in the ethical delivery of health care, none is more central than the way we envision this relationship, which has both personal and professional aspects. The way in which the physical therapist, the nurse, the radiographer, the respiratory therapist, and the physician envision their roles and functions in relation to the person they are trying to help invariably affects every moral decision made within that context.

Three general models have been suggested as descriptions of how health care workers envision their relationships with the patient. This chapter will concentrate on the social contract model and its impact on health care relations. But first we will also briefly touch on the implications of two other models for ethical decision making; the *engineering* and *paternalistic models* (Veatch, 1972).

In the engineering model the health professional abdicates his or her moral responsibility as a person in favor of leaving complete control to the patient. This model has its roots in the image of the scientist (and physician) as an objective seeker of the truth. Medical professionals who see themselves only as scientists applying the benefits of scientific research and truth feel that they must divorce themselves from all questions of values and deal only with the facts. Above all, they must remain impartial and objective. Hence, their goal is to present all the facts to the patient so that the patient can make his or her own decision. The health professional then carries out the patient's wish, whatever that might be. In this context, the health worker might help the patient commit suicide or have an abortion, even if this violated his or her own personal values. In this model, the health worker's personal values do not enter into the delivery of health care.

Veatch has three criticisms of this model. First, he argues, the idea of value-free science and medicine is a myth clearly demolished in the aftermath of the atomic mushroom clouds over Hiroshima and Nagasaki. Second, there are sit-

73

uations in health care where no matter what you do, both the decision to act and the option of doing nothing require value judgments. Third, following a model that requires a person to act against his or her conscience or at least to put conscience in neutral does not respect the autonomy and personal dignity of the health care worker.

In the paternalistic (or priestly) model, the health worker is viewed as the expert not only in medical knowledge but also in moral matters. The paternalistic health professional always knows what is best for the patient. With the health worker making all decisions, the patient must rely on the wisdom and beneficence of the expert much as a little child depends on his parents. This relationship is evident when the health worker starts off with the phrase, "Speaking as your doctor (or therapist). . . ." This model occasionally appears in news accounts. For example, someone with life-threatening gangrene may refuse amputation of both limbs "because without legs, life isn't worth anything," yet the physicians may seek a court order to force amputation because they "know what is best" for the patient.

The Contractual Relationship

In a clinic or hospital many things create distance between the patient and the health worker. Bureaucratic policies, the "red tape" of processing centers, admissions policies, insurance forms, staff shortages, computers, technological sophistications, and "machines" can interrupt communications and relationships. There is also the psychological need of health professionals to distance themselves emotionally from their patients in order to avoid "burn-out." These and other factors tend to depersonalize the relationship of patient and health professional.

The value-free engineering professional and the paternalistic health worker both have their overriding negative aspects. But both also have some good points. These desirable features have been incorporated in a third health care model, the *social contract model*. This model emphasizes the ethical need for genuine human interaction. An implied contract comes into existence when any person seeks the advice and help of another human and that other person accepts the appeal. Whether the details are verbalized or not, the sick person and the health worker enter into a contract with one another. Implicitly, they accept mutual obligations and rights. The purpose of this exercise is to clarify the moral aspects of this implicit contract by putting its main elements in writing.

Phase One

The exercise for this chapter in Part Two of this worktext contains two columns, one for the patient and one for the health care worker. You are asked to spell out the details of the implied contract between these two persons on specific issues in the ethical delivery of health care. The following are some of the details you are asked about:

1. The nature and character of the relationship—what do "genuine human interaction," "human concern," or other phrases mean in terms of the patient and health worker?

2. What obligations are accepted by the patient? By the health care worker?

3. What benefits can be expected by the patient? By the health care professional?

4. How are decision-making responsibilities handled? Is there a difference in who makes the decisions in emergency versus nonemergency situations? In everyday routine medical matters versus decisions affecting the whole plan of treatment?

5. How is the contract terminated? Who can terminate it and under what circumstances?

6. How are conflicts between the values of the professional and those of the patient handled? By compromise on the part of both? By one party abdicating responsibility as in the paternalistic or engineering models, or is there another way of resolving conflicting values?

Phase Two: Conflicting Responsibilities and Rights of the Social Contract

Conflicts between the rights and responsibilities of different persons in the health care relationship often arise, especially in areas involving the principles of autonomy, confidentiality, and truth telling. The patient has a moral right to be respected as an autonomous person: hence, he or she has a right to be fully informed about his or her condition. The health worker and others involved have a moral obligation of telling the truth and providing information necessary to allow informed consent. The patient also has a moral right to be respected as an autonomous person in the sense that what he or she reveals to the health worker must be held in confidence and not revealed to others without the patient's prior consent.

Even for physicians, with their long history of ethical codes, the question of professional confidentiality is not all that clear. The 2400-year-old Hippocratic oath speaks of the physician's knowledge gained in patient care "which on no account one must speak abroad." In the 1948 Declaration of Geneva the physician vowed, "I will hold in confidence *all* that my patient confides in me." The 1949 World Medical Association code stated that the physician "owes to his patient *absolute* secrecy on *all* which has been confided to him or which he knows because of the confidence entrusted to him."

In 1959 the British Medical Association code allowed some exception to this absolute view of confidentiality and spoke of situations where the confidence could be broken in "the best interests of the patient" even if the patient did not recognize this "best interest." In the 1960s this vague exception triggered a famous court case in Great Britain. A teenage girl living with her parents asked her physician to prescribe a contraceptive for her. Since the physician knew the young woman's parents and was their family physician, he felt obligated to inform the patient's parents without obtaining her consent. While the physician respected the broad guideline of the 1959 British Medical Association code, the daughter sued him for violation of her right to confidentiality. The British Medical Association responded by revising its code in 1971. The new code mentions two situations in which the physician may break professional confidentiality. The first is when the law requires such disclosure for the good of society. This, for instance, is the case when the law requires reporting of gunshot wounds, child abuse, or certain sexually transmitted diseases. The second exception, which is still open to interpretation, covers those situations where breaking confidentiality is in the "best interests" of the patient. If a physician believes it is in the best interests of a patient to disclose confidential information to a third party, he or she must make every effort to convince the patient to consent. If the patient refuses, the confidentiality may have to be preserved (Veatch, 1977, pp. 131–135).

In the United States the situation is very much in confusion, especially in the realm of the sexually active minor's right to confidential medical treatment. In 1983, for instance, a federal regulation was passed requiring that all health facilities receiving federal funding be required to inform in writing the parents of any minor they provided with prescription contraceptives. At the same time, 28,000 California physicians filed suit seeking an injunction against a state law that would require them to report "known or suspected sexual activity by women under 18" to their parents or legal guardians.

FOUR EXAMPLES OF CONFLICTING RIGHTS

Where would you place the balance in the conflict between the parents' right to know about medical treatment of their sexually active child because of their responsibility for that child, and the child's right to confidentiality? Circle your position on the scale of 1 to 10 below.

Child's Right to Confidentiality							Parents' Right to Know		
1	2	3	4	5	6	7	8	9	10

Explain briefly the reason for your choice.

_____

_____

_____

_____

_____

Every year 30 to 40 thousand Americans are born as a result of artificial insemination with anonymous donors' semen. In some cases the donors are very carefully screened to eliminate those with a family history of hereditary diseases. In other cases no such screening is done and the only criteria are apparent good health and general good characteristics such as average intelligence and no obvious physical defects.

What right does a child conceived by artificial insemination with donor semen have to know his or her hereditary background? Once the person considers parenthood, information about being a carrier for Tay-Sachs, sickle cell anemia, or some other hereditary disease becomes critical. Nevertheless, the donor is entitled to his anonymity. Where would you place the balance in this conflict?

Child's Right to Know							Donor's Right to Anonymity		
1	2	3	4	5	6	7	8	9	10

Explain briefly the reason for your choice.

_____

_____

_____

_____

In this conflict between the child's right to know about his or her genetic background and the donor's right to anonymity, the conflict can be resolved by not revealing the donor's identity but providing the genetic information needed.

In a second situation involving artificial insemination, this easy solution is not possible. The situation developed several years ago when a young couple in the Midwest announced their engagement.

The local physician saw the announcement and became very upset. He finally decided to call the parents of both young people into his office and break the traditional patient/physician confidentiality (Francoeur, 1977, p. 207). He informed both couples that 20 years earlier he had used the same anonymous donor to artificially inseminate both wives because of their husbands' sterility. The engaged couple were genetically half brother and sister. Having the same father, the genetic risks to any children the couple might have would be considerable. Now the dilemma: What if the parents of both the bride and the groom refuse to let the physician tell their son and daughter they have the same genetic father? Again, circle your position in the 1 to 10 continuum below:

Children's Right to Know   **Parents' Right to Confidentiality**
1   2   3   4   5   6   7   8   9   10

How would you handle the conflict of rights if one set of parents agrees to tell their child and the other set of parents refuse to allow their confidentiality to be broken?

_____

_____

_____

_____

_____

_____

_____

Our final illustration of conflicting rights involves the patient's right to know and the health worker's obligation to tell the truth. Some duty-oriented views allow no exception to the moral obligation always to tell the truth. Consequence-oriented systems can be used to defend both absolute and qualified veracity, as we saw in our first exercise. But what if providing the patient with all the information actually is harmful? Take, for example, the morality of using placebos. A physician may know that the patient is suffering from a strictly psychosomatic condition and that giving real medication is needless or harmful. Yet by prescribing a placebo and charging the regular medication price, the physician is lying to the patient. Still, telling the patient that the placebo is a powerful drug specifically designed for his condition may actually benefit the patient. As another example, what if during the initial patient/health worker contract, the patient says, "Doctor, if it's cancer, I don't want to know." Does the patient's request relieve the physician of his obligation to tell the truth? Explain your answer briefly.

_____

_____

_____

Granting that there may be some situations in which the health worker is not obliged to tell the whole truth, what general circumstances or conditions do you think might make such behavior ethical? State these conditions briefly.

_____

_____

_____

_____

_____

_____

_____

Analyzing the Ethical Implications of the Social Contract Between Patient and Health Care Worker

The first part of the exercise in Part Two gives a form for analyzing the social contract between patient and health care worker and space for you to answer the questions posed earlier. Phase Two asks you to express your views on eight sets of conflicting values or rights. Phase Three asks two questions about your own health professional code and possible guidelines for resolving conflicts of confidentiality and truth telling.

REFERENCES AND FURTHER READINGS

Barry, V. *Moral Aspects of Health Care.* Belmont, CA: Wadsworth, 1982, pp. 219–220.

Beauchamp, T.L., & Walters, L., eds. *Contemporary Issues in Bioethics,* 2nd ed. Belmont, CA: Wadsworth, 1982, pp. 198–214.

Francoeur, R.T. *Utopian Motherhood: New Trends in Human Reproduction,* 3rd ed. Cranbury, NJ: A.S. Barnes Perpetua Books, 1977, p. 287.

Fromer, M.J. *Ethical Issues in Health Care.* St. Louis: C.V. Mosby, 1981, pp. 170–182.

Gairola, G., & Skaff, K.O. Ethical reasoning in dental hygiene practice. *Dental Hygiene,* 1983, *57*(2), 16–20.

McConnell, T.C. *Moral Issues in Health Care: An Introduction to Medical Ethics.* Monterey, CA: Wadsworth Health Sciences, 1982, pp. 32–44.

Veatch, R.M. "Warning: Premarital sex may be dangerous to your health." In Veatch, R.M., ed., *Case Studies in Medical Ethics.* Cambridge, MA: Harvard University Press, 1977, pp. 131–135.

Veatch, R.M. "Models for ethical medicine in a revolutionary age." *The Hastings Center Report,* 1972, *2,* 5–7. Though derived from the physician's perspective, the models examined are relevant to all health workers.

Veatch, R.M. *A Theory of Medical Ethics.* New York: Basic Books, 1981, pp. 141–161, 296–298, 303–305. A broad-ranging, creative attempt to link the basic principles of ethical health care into a comprehensive theory, focusing on the social contract between the health worker and the patient.

NOTES

7 IDENTIFYING AND SORTING ALTERNATIVE SOLUTIONS

CHAPTER 7

IDENTIFYING AND SORTING
ALTERNATIVE SOLUTIONS

So far our steps have taken us through the broad dimensions of our world views and ethical systems, our gender-related moral development, ethical principles, and ethical rules. We then began to explore aspects of specific ethical decisions. We examined the criteria used in various triage situations of war and emergency medical care, and elements in the social contract that create new obligations for both the patient and the health worker. These steps have prepared us to explore different methods of making ethical decisions.

However, before we can make any decision on a problem case, we need to know what our options are. What solutions are open to us in this situation? What paths might we take in working out a solution to the ethical dilemmas we have identified? And how do these different options mesh with our personal and professional ethics? In this chapter we focus on identifying and sorting out the options in a particular case.

CASE STUDY: INDIGENT LATIN AMERICANS
PROVIDE REMEDY FOR BLOOD PLASMA SHORTAGE
IN THE UNITED STATES

Faced with ever-present shortages of blood plasma for surgery and transfusions, American hospitals have taken to contracting with private American companies operating blood plasma banks in Central and South American countries. These companies pay a modest fee to adults willing to sell their plasma. The clinics then sell the frozen plasma to hospitals in the United States.

Clinical Plasma Corporation, operating with a single clinic in one of the poorest Central American countries, reports that it now exports over 10,000 pints of blood plasma to the United States every month. Clinical Plasma pays its donors $5.50 per pint and reports a profit of $8.50 per pint. Critics say the company's profits are double what they claim. Company spokespersons are quick to point out their contribution to the economic recovery of the area. The company pays half a million dollars to donors annually. In an area where the average per capita income is $80 per year, regular donors can more than double or triple their incomes simply by donating plasma. Over half the donors in this clinic are unemployed or severely underemployed. In addition, the clinic employs over 100 local men and women.

The president of Clinical Plasma, an American physician and hematologist, stresses the importance his company places on maintaining the highest medical standards to protect both donors and customers who eventually receive the life-saving plasma. No one is allowed to donate plasma more than once a week, according to company policy. One in 20 volunteers is rejected because of malnutrition, anemia, or gastrointestinal diseases. Clinical Plasma's claim that its inspection procedures and quality control are equal or superior to those in the United States have been confirmed by independent outside observers.

The use of plasma donors became possible when scientists developed plasmapheresis, a way of separating protein-rich plasma from the red and white blood cells after whole blood is removed from the donor. The undamaged red and white blood cells are then returned to the donor.

The shortage of plasma in the United States is most commonly attributed to the lack of motivation among affluent Americans who are too busy to donate their plasma. The most active blood donors in America are drug addicts, alcoholics, and prisoners. This source accounts for most of the hepatitis-tainted blood that results in thousands of deaths annually in patients receiving blood transfusions. Drug usage among Clinical Plasma donors is nonexistent, and no prisoners or alcoholics are allowed to donate. Since the current test used to determine the absence of hepatitis from a blood plasma sample is only about 40% accurate, it cannot be used to eliminate donors with hepatitis. However, local FDA agents say that plasma from foreign or Mexican border clinics is less contaminated than plasma from urban American volunteers and clinics.

On the Mexico–United States border, over a dozen plasma clinics operate in much the same way as Clinical Plasma, with a few important variations. Operating in the United States places these clinics under the direct control of the Food and Drug Administration and its regulations. Donors must be at least 18, although it is easy for minors to obtain an altered Mexican identification card. In keeping with current medical opinion, volunteers are allowed to donate a pint of plasma every 72 hours. One of the seven clinics operating in El Paso has about 2,000 donors a month; the clinic pays $10 per pint and receives $25 per pint from hospitals. Most of the Texas clinics pay bonuses for repeat donors because there is less paper work with repeat donors than with new donors. Many clinics also pay donors who bring in friends who are willing to sell their plasma. The clinics advertise in both English and Spanish.

One 16-year-old interviewed admitted that he is a volunteer at least once a week. "There are 12 in my family, and it is time for me to help out in any way I can. Jobs are hard to get when you live across the border and can't get an American work permit."

Critics of the plasma clinics have argued that repeated donations raise the risk to the donor of contracting hepatitis. Some view the practice as "border vampirism," or cheap exploitation of a neighboring country, an example of American colonialism, paternalism, and indifference. Others take strong objection to Clinical Plasma, which enjoys an exclusive license in return for a surcharge tax paid to the country's military dictator.

(Adapted from "Indigent Mexicans Ready Source for Plasma at Texas Border." *The New York Times,* December 1, 1980, p. 17, and from R.M. Veatch, 1977, p. 112.)

A Warm-Up and Review on Ethical Issues and Dilemmas

Before you tackle the task of identifying the options posed by this case, practice the skills you developed in Chapters 3 and 4 by identifying basic ethical dimensions in the case described above. In the space allotted below, list specific ethical principles and rules based on those used in earlier chapters. Then, check your list against the questions in the paragraph below your answers.

YOUR LIST OF ETHICAL PRINCIPLES, ISSUES, AND GUIDELINES

SOME THOUGHTS ABOUT THE ABOVE
ETHICAL INSIGHTS

- Volunteering to donate blood for the benefit of others has normally been thought of as an altruistic act, a charitable recognition of the needs of others. Do the plasma clinics violate this personal ethic? If so, to what extent?

- To what extent should efficiency in meeting the needs of Americans be used as an argument in deciding the ethics of this situation?

- To what extent does this practice depersonalize the donor? Or is this depersonalization relative, being balanced by the improved quality of life enjoyed by the donor who thereby doubles or triples his or her annual income?

- To what extent is commercialization morally acceptable in health care delivery?

- Are these clinics within the range of ethical compromise necessary to save lives and meet our desperate need for plasma?

- Is it more ethical to close these clinics to avoid exploiting the poor, leaving them with their substandard income and allowing hundreds of thousands to die for want of plasma? Or is it more ethical to keep the clinics open, improve the quality of life of the poor, save hundreds of thousands of lives, and allow private business its profit?

- What other ethical principles do you find applicable to this case? Did you list any ethical issues not mentioned above?

IDENTIFYING OPTIONS

For the first phase of this step, ignore the ethical issues and all consequences. Simply list every option you can think of as a way of handling this situation.

Two options are often overlooked in such a list, although both are obvious. The first option in any list can be to do nothing, or leave things as they are. In this case, doing nothing would mean permitting the clinics to continue their business as they have been. The second obvious option can be to stop whatever is going on, in this case, to close down all plasma clinics and not to allow any such business to operate within the United States.

On a separate page, list as many other options as you can uncover. Then compare your list with the list of options below.

Remember for this initial phase to ignore all ethical issues and all consequences, good or bad, of each option. Just list every option you can think of. In our later steps we will use the four boxes at the end of each option to sort out the more ethical options and eliminate others.

Phase One: A List of Options for Plasma Clinics

	Violates Professional Code	Violates Personal Ethics	Optimizes Values	Promotes Interest

1. Allow the clinics to continue operating as they are.

2. Close all clinics immediately and enact laws prohibiting such businesses in the United States.

   Beyond these two alternatives, one can devise a wide range of variations on the single general alternative of allowing the clinics to continue operating, but under certain new conditions. Each new condition can constitute a separate alternative. Thus,

3. Keep the clinics open but have tighter security on donor identification, either fingerprints or photographic ID cards, to keep minors from donating.

4. Keep the clinics open but stop the policy of paying donors.

5. Increase pretesting of donors for hepatitis.

6. Identify origin of plasma and allow the potential recipient to say whether he or she is willing to risk use of such plasma.

7. Prohibit payment of bonuses for repeat donors.

8. Prohibit bonuses for bringing in new donors.

9. Prohibit all bonuses for repeat donors and bringing in new donors.

10. Double the standard payment to donors and at the same time restrict the frequency one can donate.

	Violates Professional Code	Violates Personal Ethics	Optimizes Values	Promotes Interest
11. Include statement of hazards involved in repeated plasma donation in all clinic advertisements.				
12. Prohibit advertising in Spanish.				
13. Allow clinics operating within U.S. boundaries to accept plasma only from proven American citizens.				
14. Require clinics to provide or pay for free hepatitis treatment if a donor contracts the disease.				
15. Allow repeat donations only after specific long intervals—once a month, once every three months, twice a year, or even only once a year.				
16. Enact a donor surcharge tax on the clinics to pay for developing a new, reliable, and safe hepatitis vaccine or treatment.				
17. Require clinics to provide complete physical examinations and nutrition counseling for their repeat donors.				
18. Require clinics to be operated only by federal or state agencies, and not as private corporations interested in profit for their stockholders.				
19. Prohibit the operation of any plasma clinic within 100 miles of U.S. territorial boundaries, to reduce the number of aliens able to donate.				
20. Have federal or state regulation of clinics' payments to donors and the fees charged hospitals or physicians for such plasma.				
21. Require stricter standards than currently in effect to reduce the chance of donors getting hepatitis, even at the risk of being overly cautious.				

	Violates Professional Code	Violates Personal Ethics	Optimizes Values	Promotes Interest

22. Require strict training of staff and frequent inspection to assure the highest standards of hygiene and patient safety.

23. Provide an environment that is more personalized and less commercial than current clinical settings.

24. Provide interviews and counseling by clinics and/or independent agencies to ascertain how the foreign donors react to this opportunity and to learn how the operation could be improved or made more personal and less "exploitative."

25. Provide the equivalent of food stamps in return for plasma donations instead of monetary payment.

26. Where more than one clinic operates within a 50 or 100 mile radius, establish a communications network to prevent one person from donating at two different clinics before a safe time has elapsed.

27. Maintain accurate epidemiologic records on individual clinics and close down those that have an unacceptable hepatitis rate.

28. Trace contaminated plasma to the donor and provide free hepatitis treatment to affected donors.

29. Stop all payments for plasma and develop an educational program to promote voluntarism among Americans to meet the need for plasma.

30. Give high priority to research funding to develop an inexpensive, safe artificial plasma and then close down the clinic, or use a surcharge on the clinics to fund such research.

Violates Professional Code	Violates Personal Ethics	Optimizes Values	Promotes Interest

31. Prohibit such clinics within the United States but allow hospitals to purchase plasma from clinics run by or approved by foreign governments within their territories.

How complete do you think this list is? Can you think of another option not listed here?

The above list of 31 options is the result of combined student efforts in several years of biomedical ethics classes. Yet it is not complete. There is at least one more option that can be added. More important, this new option contains some interesting solutions to the ethical dilemmas posed by the case. It would be possible to close all the clinics and pass a federal law requiring every American citizen over 18 to donate at least 1 pint of blood plasma annually. Those who have valid religious or medical reasons against donating would be exempted. Such a law could completely eliminate the need for the foreign blood plasma clinics.

Phase Two: Elimination of Unethical Alternatives

Return to the list of specific ethical issues you identified for this case in the warm-up section on page 85. Refresh your memory on the principles and guidelines you listed there. Then, in the first column of boxes to the right of each alternative, check those alternatives that you find are in contradiction to your professional code.

In the second column of boxes, check any alternative that violates your personal ethics.

Eliminate these unacceptable options by crossing out those checked as unacceptable to you either professionally or personally.

Phase Three: Clustering of Alternatives According to Interest Groups

With this reduced list of ethically acceptable options, you can further simplify your choices by clustering the alternatives in terms of specific interest groups.

Read through your remaining options to find those alternatives that optimize or promote the ethical principles (guidelines) you identified as important in this case. When you find an alternative that relates in a positive way to an ethical issue, enter the number you assigned that individual concern in the warm-up on page 85 in the third box opposite the appropriate alternative.

A final step in sorting out the remaining alternatives involves clustering the options you find especially attractive. First, ask yourself which of the options that you did not cross out as professionally or personally unacceptable promotes the interests and concerns of

1. Donors

2. Clinics and their owners

3. Ultimate beneficiaries, the patients who receive the plasma in transfusions

Enter the number of the affected interest group (1, 2, and 3) appropriate to each remaining alternative in the fourth box.

Next, pick out all the options that promote or optimize a particular ethical concern or interest group. See if some of the options overlap, complement, or reinforce one another. Can two or more alternatives be effectively combined into a single new alternative that is stronger and more positive than the same individual alternatives taken separately? Cluster your remaining options in this reduced list.

These options can then be used with any of the decision-making methods outlined in the remaining chapters and exercises of this text. However, we will not be pursuing this case any further. The remaining chapters will pick up new cases to illustrate individual decision methods. Do keep in mind that the technique used here to demonstrate the identification and sorting of options is an essential step in any decision-making process you may use.

Applying This Exercise to Your Case Study

Now that you have gone through this exercise step by step, you can develop your skills by using the same method with a case of your own choice, or with a case assigned to you in class. You can use the standard form for identifying and sorting out alternatives in the exercise in Part Two.

REFERENCES AND FURTHER READINGS

Easton, A. *Decision Making: A Short Course in Problem Solving for Professionals.* Translate objectives into criteria and identify all feasible alternatives, Part III, Step 4, pp. 1–33. New York: John Wiley & Sons, 1976.

Hill, P.H. et al. *Making Decisions: A Multidisciplinary Introduction.* Reading, MA: Addison-Wesley, 1979, pp. 23–24.

Veatch, R.M. "Blood money." In Veatch, R.M., *Case Studies in Medical Ethics.* Cambridge, MA: Harvard University Press, 1977, p. 112.

NOTES

8 THE OPERATIONAL DECISION TECHNIQUE

CHAPTER 8
THE OPERATIONAL DECISION TECHNIQUE

No matter how much you know about a case study, you will never have all the information you would like or think you need to make a good decision. Some critical information will always be missing. Despite this, you will have to make a decision.

When 21-year-old Karen Anne Quinlan was admitted to the emergency room at Newton Memorial Hospital the night of April 15, 1975, she was in a life-threatening coma. She had ceased breathing for at least two 15-minute periods and had received some mouth-to-mouth resuscitation from friends at a party. Her temperature was 100°F, and she appeared unresponsive to her environment. In the crisis atmosphere of the emergency room and the rush to find a neurologist for consultation, critical time passed during which those close to Karen Anne at the time she went into her coma forgot some crucial details that might have led to different decisions. Later, the New Jersey Supreme Court stated that "the history at the time of her admission to that hospital was *essentially incomplete and uninformative.*"

The decision was made to perform a tracheotomy and to put Karen Anne on a ventilator. Five days later, when she was transferred to the intensive care unit at St. Clare's Hospital in nearby Denville, New Jersey, that missing information was lost forever. Karen Anne was in cycles of waking and sleeping. Although she could blink, grimace, and cry out, she was "totally unaware of anyone or anything around her."

Yet the neurologist, a consulting pulmonary specialist, and the respiratory therapist at St. Clare's had to make new decisions about the medical options open to them and the most ethical way to handle Karen's coma. Meanwhile, the same missing information affected Karen Anne's parents as they waivered in their decision of whether or not they wanted to have the ventilator and feeding through a nasogastric tube continued. During this time, everyone involved with the case felt totally exasperated by the crucial missing information.

When the court allowed the physician and respiratory therapist to wean Karen Anne from the ventilator and transfer her to a nursing home, few expected her to live. She was in a grotesque, fetal-like posture and had lost 40 pounds. Her muscles were rigid and deformed, leaving her in a "chronic and persistent vegetative state.'' Yet in late 1983 she was still alive, though her coma continues as deep as ever (Branson et al., 1976).

No matter whether a case study contains two paragraphs, two pages, 20 pages, or volumes, the information is always limited. Medical experts have offered scholarly analyses of the Quinlan case. Ethicists have debated the case. The lawyers and courts have argued the issues. Books have been written. Still, 8 years later, we lack certain information about the origin and circumstances of Karen Anne's coma, information that many feel is crucial. Yet at each step, health care professionals had to make decisions; the only recourse was to make an operational decision. Using all the information available at the time and calling on their experience and ethical sensitivity, the professionals in the Quinlan case made their decisions.

Most decisions made in the delivery of health care and in medical ethics are operational, or working, decisions based on the facts at hand and subject to modification or even reversal when additional facts become known. These decisions are made as thoughtfully and responsibly as possible with the information we have, but their provisional nature becomes evident in the new information and new perspective another day brings. That is the human situation: we make our operational decision today as best we can, act on it, and hope tomorrow's insights do not prove us wrong. If they do, we humbly admit that we made what we now know from hindsight to have been a mistake. Hopefully, we can compensate for what has proved to be the wrong decision.

In this exercise, as in all the subsequent exercises, you will deal with limited information. A brief case study is provided as an example and worked through using a particular decision technique. In this chapter, the case is that of a 75-year-old physician with Parkinson's disease who asks his best friend to be with him while he commits suicide. In working with this case, you will face the reality of limited information coupled with the need to make an operational decision as to whether the friend can morally participate in the physician's suicide.

CASE STUDY: A MAN SUPPORTS HIS FRIEND IN HIS DECISION TO COMMIT SUICIDE

At the Tenth Annual Euthanasia Educational Council conference in New York City, Morgan Sibbert, a retired engineer, shared his experience with a concerned audience of over 200. His physician friend of 39 years, Wallace Proctor, had decided to commit suicide. At age 75, Proctor had Parkinson's disease, a debilitating disease with tremors and muscular rigidity caused by degeneration of the basal ganglia in the brain.

Several years ago the two friends had discussed Proctor's illness and the circumstances under which one might be morally justified in ending one's life. At that time, Mr. Sibbert and his wife were able to persuade their friend that his disease was still not interfering seriously with his quality of life. In subsequent years, as the disease progressed, and particularly after a recent heart attack, Dr. Proctor brought up the question again.

Sibbert admitted that his friend "could take the pills himself, no problem there. But to give him the comfort and the peace of being with a friend in his last days and to make sure that he was not thwarted, this was very important. He came to me because I was a friend, and because I would guard his right to do this—that was my most important function."

Dr. Proctor's wife, Maria, would not share in this decision since it required her "to look the other way," something she, as a nurse, could not accept. Also, in Proctor's home state of Colorado, suicide and aiding in a suicide are criminal acts. Since suicide is not a criminal offense in Pennsylvania, Sibbert invited his friend to visit him at his home in Swarthmore, Pennsylvania. With both wives traveling on business, the two men could be alone together. Dr. Proctor welcomed the invitation because he was concerned that if his suicide was a criminal act and his friend were involved, there would be delays in removing his brain, which he wanted donated for medical research on Parkinson's disease.

There were many details for the men to work out together. Arrangements were made to take Dr. Proctor's brain to the University of Pennsylvania hospital for an immediate postmortem autopsy. Dr. Proctor wrote to family members and arranged his will. But the two friends also relaxed, filling their time with laughter and reminiscences of their 39 years as friends.

On August 16, Dr. Proctor remarked at dinner that this was their last meal together. That night he took a lethal dose of Seconal.

Commenting on Mr. Sibbert's experience, Dr. Joseph Fletcher, a pioneer in the field of medical ethics and the president of the Society for the Right to Die, noted that "the moral question which still hangs on is whether we may not only let a patient die rather than prolong the patient's life, but whether we may do something directly to hasten the patient's end."

(Adapted from a *New York Times* report by C. Gerald Fraser, Dec. 11, 1977, p. 47.)

A Warm-Up and Review on Ethical Issues and Principles

Before you tackle this exercise in reaching an operational decision, review the ethical principle and issues related to autonomy discussed in Chapter 3. Use the following questions to sharpen your understanding of these values in this case. These can be discussed in class before moving on to Phase One below.

- In your view, is helping someone commit suicide the same as homicide?

- Does the sanctity-of-life ethic, in the duty-oriented natural law system, require that all human life be preserved at any cost, or does the quality of life take precedence over mere physical survival?

- Is Dr. Proctor's wife right in her view that as a nurse, whose primary obligation is to preserve life, it would be immoral for her to approve or abet her husband's suicide?

- Should society have the right to intervene in order to protect individuals from themselves even when they do not want to continue living? Or should society allow or facilitate a person to end his or her life when the pain being suffered becomes intolerable?

- If we are morally bound to reduce pain and suffering in this world, is there a moral difference between allowing terminally ill persons to die peacefully and accelerating their dying in order to relieve pain? Does your answer change when you add to this question a belief in a life hereafter?

- Is death with dignity morally more preferable to physical survival for a few extra days or months?

- Is the direct taking of a human life ever permissible, or is God the only one to decide when a person dies, since He is life's author? How does this issue affect an atheist or humanist who does not believe in a supreme being?

- What impact will the growing number of older persons with degenerative diseases have on our understanding of the moral values of human life and good health?

- What moral values come into play as we improve our technological ability to extend life? What are considered "ordinary efforts" or "extraordinary means" of preserving life?

These questions can be related to the principle of autonomy—our moral obligation to respect an autonomous person, his or her choices, and the freedom to act on those considered choices. They also raise questions about less general ethical issues, such as the issues of human worth or the sanctity of human life. While it is permissible to allow someone to die without attempting heroic measures, is human life so valuable that it is never morally permissible to kill oneself or another person? One can also ask questions about the values and disvalues of suicide for the person contemplating it and for the family.

MAKING AN OPERATIONAL DECISION

Which of the five options below is most acceptable to you? Can you suggest a more ethical option? Circle the option you personally prefer or the one most acceptable to the class as a whole.

1. Participate in and support Proctor's suicide.

2. Refuse to participate and persuade his wife to have him committed as mentally incompetent.

3. Refuse to participate and do nothing to inform Proctor's wife of his intention.

4. Refuse to participate but warn Proctor's wife.

5. Your option, to _____.

Explain briefly why you or the class selected this option.

_____

_____

_____

_____

_____

Phase One: Factors Most Influencing Your Choice of Option

Think again about your choice of option. What particular factors or consequences played the strongest role in your selection? What were you most concerned about? Pick the three most important factors for you or for the class. Indicate these with a 1, 2, or 3 in the space before the appropriate factors below.

1. ____ *Economic* factors—the cost to the tax payer, the cost to the hospital in terms of available but limited facilities and professional staff, the cost to Dr. Proctor's family, the effect of suicide on Dr. Proctor's insurance, and so on.

2. ____ *Legal* considerations—in this case, the differences in Colorado and Pennsylvania laws, the legal consequences for Mr. Sibbert, the need for better federal or state laws, and so on.

3. ____ *Social* considerations—the effect of legalized euthanasia or mercy killing

on society, our constitutional concept of human life and rights, the value and respect our society accords older persons, and so on.

4. ____ *Political* factors—the effects of the option chosen on our political system.

5. ____ *Personal* considerations—the relationship of the option chosen to personal rights, autonomy, integrity, privacy, and personal values.

6. ____ *Religious and/or ethical* considerations—moral, religious, philosophical, or ethical positions on the issues of euthanasia, mercy killing, and suicide.

7. ____ *Medical* considerations—the consequences of legalizing or prohibiting euthanasia on the different health care professionals: physicians, nurses, allied health personnel, social workers, and counselors.

8. ____ *Technical* considerations—the effects of this particular case and of ones similar to it on scientific or medical research and the continued advance of basic research, and possible or likely effects on the psychology of researchers and health care professionals in general.

9. ____ *Other factors* or considerations not listed above. State briefly:

_____

_____

_____

_____

Share your views of the three most important factors with the rest of the class or with a friend to compare viewpoints. Is there any agreement on your influential factors? Complete the chart below listing the number of students choosing each factor as their first, second, or third choice.

Factor Ranking	First	Second	Third
Economic			
Legal			
Social			
Political			
Personal			
Religious			
Technical			
Other			

EXPLANATION OF THREE MAIN FACTORS
IN YOUR CHOICE

In discussing with the class or analyzing on your own the influence of the above factors on your choice of option, try to summarize your ideas about the three key factors in brief concise statements.

Indicate your most influential factor and give your explanation.

_____

_____

_____

_____

_____

_____

_____

_____

_____

Indicate your second most influential factor and give your explanation.

_____

_____

_____

_____

_____

_____

_____

_____

_____

_____

_____

_____

Indicate your third most influential factor and give your explanation.

_____

_____

_____

_____

_____

_____

_____

If you or the class found that personal factors were most influential in your decision supporting Sibbert's action, your reasons might include the following: Dr. Proctor should have the final decision about his life and future. He has lived a full, rich life. The prospect of slowly "rotting away" is not acceptable to him. He is not irrational or out of his mind; he discussed the possibility of suicide several years ago, and now feels that the disease has reached the point where his quality of life no longer makes life worth living. He has taken care of his family responsibility and is not acting on impulse. Mr. Sibbert's personal decision to comfort his old friend appears to be in keeping with the personal values of both.

If you or the class selected an option disapproving Sibbert's action, you might have felt that Dr. Proctor should have the right of self-determination, but this does not mean that his friend should help him commit suicide. You may have reasoned that no matter how rational the decision, it is bound to have emotional and psychological consequences for Dr. Proctor's wife and family. His wife has already indicated she cannot accept his decision. Self-preservation is a basic human drive; suicide is never a rational, sane choice.

If one of your factors was religious, you might have favored Sibbert's acceptance because you did not want to impose your morality on another person whose religious or philosophical outlook accepts a rational decision of suicide. Your reasons might have included the following: We have to respect the rights of a person who believes in a life hereafter and decides to end his or her life because of its quality, the endless pain, and the dependency. For centuries, natural selection killed off people like Dr. Proctor long before their lives and diseases became unbearable. Now, modern medicine has reduced "survival of the fittest," and is playing God by keeping people alive. Since we have replaced natural selection with human selection, we have the moral right to end a life that "nature" would have ended if our medicine had not intervened. When the future is hopeless and endless pain, the quality of life is more important than the length of one's life.

But you might also have opposed Sibbert's cooperation on the grounds that since only God can give life, only He should take it. Taking one's own life is always immoral. Encouraging someone's suicide by participating in it is just as immoral as taking one's own life.

Share your views and discuss them with members of the class, in pairs or in small groups. Question the explanations to find out what other people think, especially if their views differ from yours. The point is not to argue or convince but to learn from others.

Phase Two: Outside Consultation

In some ethical dilemmas you have time to consult with others. If you had time to consult with others about how to handle Dr. Proctor's planned suicide, with whom—besides Proctor and Sibbert—would you like to consult before making your decision? Check those you would want to talk to.

1. Proctor's wife, Maria

2. Proctor's children

3. Clergy or religious leader

4. Psychologist

5. Specialist in suicide and crisis intervention

6. Health professionals who deal with the terminally ill

7. Lawyer

8. Advocates of rational suicide

9. Other _____

Explain briefly your reasons for wanting this consultation.

_____

_____

_____

_____

_____

_____

_____

Phase Three: No Outside Consultation Possible

The circumstances in our case may make outside consultation impossible. We may have to reach an immediate decision. But perhaps we can get more information from those mentioned in our case. If you had only the above information in our case and were allowed to talk at length with only one of the three persons in the case, would you choose to talk with Dr. Proctor, his wife, or Mr. Sibbert? What information do you think this person could provide that might influence your decision?

_____

_____

_____

_____

_____

_____

_____

Phase Four: Policy Decisions

As a part of your operational decision you might want to consider your views about establishing some sort of standard public policy, on the federal or state level or for the affected institution or community, to cover situations such as our sample case. You might also want to consider the advantages of not establishing any policy. Should we have laws prohibiting or regulating suicide, or is every situation so unique that it has to be decided on its own merits by the parties involved? Which of the following approaches do you favor?

1. A national policy such as a federal law that would either decriminalize or prohibit suicide. Would such a law provide guidelines to protect the individual's right to self-determination? Would such a law also prevent abuse and exploitation by relatives of the aged, handicapped, and terminally ill persons of all ages?

2. State laws rather than federal laws, even though different states might have different laws and policies.

3. No legal restrictions, with the decision being left to the individual and his or her family and health care team. This would include no restrictions on "how-to" guide books for rational suicide.

Explain briefly the reasons for your position.

_____

_____

_____

_____

_____

_____

_____

_____

_____

Phase Five: Crucial Missing Information

In the final step of our operational decision, reexamine your case and pick out one detail or specific bit of information not included in the case study that might alter or influence your decision. What information that you do not have would you want before making your operational decision? Examples might be more information about Parkinson's disease and the extent of its effects on Dr. Proctor at this time, the likely psychological consequences to Proctor's family, his financial (insurance) arrangements, his religious beliefs, or whether Proctor would go ahead if he did not have Sibbert's support. You may add your own examples below.

_____

_____

_____

_____

_____

_____

Applying This Exercise to Your Case Study

Now that you have gone through this operational decision exercise step by step with our sample case, you can polish your skills by using this technique with a case of your own choice or with a case assigned to you in class. An exercise in this approach can be found in Part Two of this worktext.

REFERENCES AND FURTHER READINGS

Annas, G. "In re Quinlan: Legal comfort for doctors." *Hastings Center Report*, 1976, 6(3), pp. 29–31.

Barry, V. *Moral Aspects of Health Care.* Belmont, CA: Wadsworth, 1982, pp. 397–430.

Branson, R., et al. "The Quinlan decision: Five commentaries." *Hastings Center Report*, 1976, 6(1), pp. 8–23.

Easton, A. *Decision Making: A Short Course in Problem Solving for Professionals.* Initiating the Decision Process. Part II, Steps 1–3, pp. 1–43. New York: John Wiley & Sons, 1976.

Hill, P.H., et al. *Making Decisions: A Multidisciplinary Introduction.* Reading, MA: Addison-Wesley, 1979.

Janis, I.L., & Mann, L. *Decision Making: A Psychological Analysis of Conflict, Choice and Commitment.* New York: Free Press, 1977.

McConnell, T.C. *Moral Issues in Health Care: An Introduction to Medical Ethics.* Monterey, CA: Wadsworth Health Sciences, 1982, pp. 72–73, 130–137, 151–157.

Policy Research Incorporated and the Center for Technology Assessment, New Jersey Institute of Technology. *A Comprehensive Study of the Ethical, Legal, and Social Implications of Advances in Biomedical and Behavioral Research and Technology.* Baltimore: Policy Research Inc., 1975. The central exercise in Chapter 8 is based on a Policy Evaluation Instrument in this study mandated by the National Commission for the Protection of Human Subjects of Biomedical and Behavioral Research.

Powledge, T.M., & Steinfels, P. "Following the news on Karen Quinlan." *Hastings Center Report*, 1975, 5(6), pp. 5–6, 28.

NOTES

9 COSTS AND BENEFITS OF AN ALTERNATIVES BALANCE SHEET

CHAPTER 9
COSTS AND BENEFITS OF AN ALTERNATIVES BALANCE SHEET

Every option we face in resolving a problem has its inherent costs and benefits, some positive consequences along with several negative consequences. The Janus-like character of alternatives is a reality we need to face and resolve. Using an alternatives balance sheet is one way to analyze the positive and negative consequences of several relatively acceptable options in a case. By weighing the pros and cons of each alternative we can reach a decision on the most ethical option.

In this chapter we work through the case of parents who disagree on the fate of their 12-year-old son. There are only two alternatives, which simplifies our sample: the mother wants to continue the life-support systems, whereas the father favors discontinuing life-support and allowing nature to take its course.

CASE STUDY: PARENTS DISAGREE OVER FATE OF "BRAIN DEATH" SON

On July 2, 1978, 12-year-old Larry Thompson was shot in the heart by an air-powered, pellet-firing rifle that his father, Louis, was oiling. The father, a 49-year-old clerk, was distraught over the shooting, which police listed as accidental.

By August 15, physicians disagreed among themselves whether Larry, whose life was being maintained by a respirator, had suffered total brain death. One physician stated that nerve cell activity was the only one of six medically recognized criteria of life still evidenced by Larry. The other five criteria were completely negative, indicating that Larry's brain was no longer functioning. Since the parents could not agree on continuing the life support systems, the hospital asked its lawyer to seek a court ruling on what to do. After listening to the medical testimony, Sussex Probate Court Judge Jeremiah Rutkowski ruled that the youth "still had nerve cell activity and should be considered alive."

"He'll never be the same," the father reacted. "I'd like the plug pulled. He's a vegetable, and I can't live seeing him like that." (Earlier, Larry's father had told the court and physicians that he wanted the life-support systems continued, in hope of a "miracle.")

The youth's mother, Jane, disagreed with her husband and wanted the support systems continued: "My mind understands but my heart prays for a miracle!"

Six weeks after the accident, physicians on the case agreed with outside experts that chances of a "miracle recovery" were less than one in a million.

The judge then had to rule on whether to allow treatment to be discontinued or to order it continued.

(Adapted from reports in local Massachusetts newspapers. Names have been changed.)

First Option: The judge should order the physicians to continue life-support so long as one of the six criteria is positive. This was the mother's choice.

Second Option: The judge should allow physicians to stop treatment since five of the six commonly accepted criteria indicate that Larry has suffered irreversible "brain death." This was the father's choice.

Phase One

In this exercise, each option is treated independently until you reach the end and analyze your results. Your first task is to identify as many positive and negative consequences as you can for option 1, continuing treatment. You should list all options regardless of whether they have a high or low moral character. (The ethical content and relative weight of your consequences will be sorted out in Phase Two of this exercise.) The following list includes some of the **positive consequences** you might identify for continuing the life support system.

	Ethical Importance	General Weight
1. He may come out of coma and recover.		
2. Father avoids the guilt feelings of having "pulled the plug."		
3. Medical research on comas may be furthered.		
4. Avoids the responsibility of "playing God."		
5. Father could be charged with homicide if son dies.		

	Ethical Importance	General Weight
6. Avoids legal complications for hospital and physicians.		
7. Publicity of physicians' efforts may bring grant money to the hospital.		

What other positive consequences of this option can you identify? Add these to the above list. If you do not think some of the consequences cited above are realistic, cross them out.

The following are among the **negative consequences** you might identify.

	Ethical Importance	General Weight
1. Increases family's financial burden.		
2. Prolongs emotional stress for parents.		
3. Requires continuous use of manpower and equipment for the hospital.		
4. Has a negative effect on family's other children.		
5. Father may divorce mother over disagreement and mother may not be able to handle added emotional and financial strain.		
6. Costs taxpayers if family and insurance cannot cover bills.		
7. Other patients with better prognoses for recovery may be deprived of needed treatment.		

What other negative consequences can you identify for this first option? Add these to the above list, and cross out those consequences you do not find realistic.

Now repeat this same process for your second option. The following list includes **positive consequences** you might identify for discontinuing life-support.

	Ethical Importance	General Weight
1. Permits death with dignity.		
2. Parents face responsibility for son's death.		
3. Father avoids continual reminder.		
4. Medical expense ended.		
5. Hospital saves money.		
6. Saves son pain if he can still sense it.		
7. Hospital can work with patients with better chances for recovery.		
_____		
_____		
_____		
_____		

Add any other positive consequences you can think of and cross out consequences you consider unrealistic.

The following are among the **negative consequences** you might identify.

	Ethical Importance	General Weight
1. Violates sanctity of life.		
2. Removes even remote chance of recovery.		
3. May create legal problems for father if he consents.		
4. Hampers research on comas.		
5. Parents have to accept responsibility.		

	Ethical Importance	General Weight
6. Physicians have to acknowledge "defeat."		
7. Hospital and physicians may be sued.		
_____		
_____		
_____		
_____		

Add any other negative consequences you can think of and cross out any consequences you consider unrealistic.

Phase Two

After listing all the positive and negative consequences you can think of for each alternative, the next task is to determine the importance of each of these consequences by assigning each a relative weight on a scale of 1 to 5. Take the first list of consequences on page 110. Examine the seven positive consequences and whatever additional consequences you found. Ignoring for the moment the ethical dimensions, pick out the most important consequence(s) and give it a weight of 5. Then pick out the least important negative outcome(s) and give it a weight of 1. Write these ratings in the column titled General Weight. Rate the rest of your negative consequences between 1 and 5, depending on your judgment of their general importance. Use the following weighting scale:

5 = Very important

4 = Important

3 = Worth considering

2 = Of minor importance

1 = Of very minor importance

Repeat this process for the three remaining lists, weighting each consequence but ignoring the moral aspects.

Next, repeat this weighting process with the consequences in the four lists, but this time focus on the moral or ethical issues. Ignore those legal, social, psychological, economic, or technical consequences that have no ethical or moral character. Using the same 1 to 5 weighting scale you just used, assign a weight to each of the consequences that relate to ethical or moral issues. Write the rating in the column titled Ethical Importance.

When you have finished this double weighting of the consequences, add up the general importance weights you assigned to the positive consequences of the first option on page 110. Enter that total in the table below. Add up the ethical importance weights for this same list and enter it below. Repeat this process for the negative consequences and enter the totals below.

ALTERNATIVES BALANCE SHEET SUMMARY

	General Weight	Ethical Importance
First option: Positive consequences		
Negative consequences		

The balance of ethical weights for this first option favors which set of consequences? (Circle one.)   POSITIVE   NEGATIVE

By how many points? (Subtract negative total from positive total.) _____

	General Weight	Ethical Importance
Second option: Positive consequences		
Negative consequences		

The balance of ethical weights for this second option favors which set of outcomes? (Circle one.)   POSITIVE   NEGATIVE
By how many points? _____

Which option has the *highest positive balance?* (Circle one.)   Option 1
Option 2

If the ethical balance for one alternative is strongly positive and the balance for the second option is strongly negative, you have resolved the problem. If the two balances are both positive, you can reexamine them to make sure that the strongest positive ethical balance is, in effect, really the strongest. (If you have only two options, as in our sample case, then a positive ethical balance for one option should be matched by a negative ethical balance for the other option.)

If two positive ethical balances are very close, you may have to reexamine the weight you gave each consequence. In the end, your balances may be too close for the difference to be significant. In this case, you may have to use another decision technique. If your ethical balances for both options are strongly negative, you may want to look for a different alternative you had not previously identified.

Look now at the totals for general importance weights. Is the option with the highest positive consequence total for ethical importance the same option with the highest general weight? If your ethical values favor one option and the economic, legal, technical, and other nonmoral balance favors a different option, which way do you go? Explain briefly below.

Phase Three

This step is useful as a check when you analyze your case with the alternatives balance sheet in this chapter and either the operational decision technique in the previous chapter or the decisional matrix in Chapter 11.

If you have used these different approaches with the same case, your conclusion from the alternatives balance sheet may agree with your conclusion from either the operational decision exercise or the decision matrix. In this event, you have a confirmation of your analysis and decision.

If, on the other hand, your conclusions are in conflict, you should try to decide why conflict exists. That challenge can itself give you a new insight into the problem and hopefully a more satisfying answer. Remember, none of these techniques is guaranteed. Their usefulness and success depend on the thoughtfulness and effort you apply. Some techniques work better with certain cases than with others, and depending on the case, some techniques may on occasion by useless. Knowing which approach works best with which type of case is a matter of experience with the different approaches.

Applying This Exercise to Your Case Study

Now that you have completed an alternatives balance sheet step by step with a sample case, you can develop your skill in this approach to decision making using a case of your own choice, or a case assigned to you in class. You can use the standard form for this exercise, which you will find in Part Two of this worktext.

If you select your own case, you will need to identify the different options open to you and to select two or three for analysis using the balance sheets. If your instructor assigns you a case for analysis, your options may already be spelled out for you, or you may have to identify the two or three alternatives you want to analyze with the balance sheets.

REFERENCES AND FURTHER READINGS

Baram, M.S. "Cost-benefit analysis: An inadequate basis for health, safety, and environmental regulatory decision making." In Beauchamp, T.L., & Walters, L., eds. *Contemporary Issues in Bioethics*, 2nd ed. Belmont, CA: Wadsworth, 1982.

Beauchamp, T.L., & Childress, J.F. *Principles of Biomedical Ethics.* New York: Oxford University Press, 1979, pp. 119, 136, 145–153.

Easton, A. *Decision Making: A Short Course in Problem Solving for Professionals.* Part 4, Step 5: Predict and quantify outcomes of alternatives on all criteria; Part 5, Steps 6 and 7: Translate outcome scores into value scores and weight criteria; and Part VI, Step 8: Select a rule and compute the best alternative. New York: John Wiley & Sons, 1976.

Fuchs, V.R. "What is cost-benefit analysis?" In Beauchamp, T.L., & Walters, L., eds. *Contemporary Issues in Bioethics*, 2nd ed. Belmont, CA: Wadsworth, 1982.

Janis, I.L., & Mann, L. *Decision Making: A Psychological Analysis of Conflict, Choice and Commitment.* New York: Free Press, 1977, pp. 135–170, 377–379, 405–410.

Kieffer, G.H. *Bioethics: A Textbook of Issues.* Reading, MA: Addison-Wesley, 1979, pp. 121–122, 134, 155.

Policy Research Incorporated and the Center for Technology Assessment, New Jersey Institute of Technology. *A Comprehensive Study of the Ethical, Legal, and Social Implications of Advances in Biomedical and Behavioral Research and Technology.* Baltimore: Policy Research Inc., 1975. The central exercise in Chapter 9 is based on a policy evaluation instrument in this study mandated by the National Commission for the Protection of Human Subjects of Biomedical and Behavioral Research.

Purtillo, R.B., & Cassel, C.K. *Ethical Dimensions in the Health Professions.* Philadelphia: W.B. Saunders, 1981, p. 210.

NOTES

10 THE DECISION TREE TECHNIQUE

CHAPTER 10
THE DECISION TREE TECHNIQUE

In making decisions, most people try in some informal way to weigh the alternatives open to them based on their expected immediate or short-term results. The decision tree format, commonly used in business management, has an advantage because it structures and makes explicit some elements in the decision process that are implicit but not often examined carefully in less structured techniques. In a decision tree you draw a picture to visualize three important factors. As a first step you identify the alternatives. Then you assign probability estimates to the events associated with each alternative. Finally, you calculate the pay-off, or consequences, for each combination of a decision or action and its immediate results. When you finish you have what looks very much like a tree lying on its side, with branches spreading out to the right from a single trunk or starting point on the left.

Each branching point in the tree represents one of two kinds of points, or nodes, indicated by a square or circle. The starting point where you make a decision or act is represented by a small square with branches to the right listing all the relevant decisions or actions you might take. Only two alternatives are given for the example used here, to medicate or not to medicate. But, as we discovered in Chapter 7, a case may have many alternatives. In this situation, your list of alternatives or possible decisions depends a lot on your creativity, insight, and past experiences. The more creative you are, the more complete your decision tree will be. Also remember that taking no action, as we do in the case here, is a perfectly acceptable alternative.

The second kind of branching point or node, shown as a small circle, indicates the chance events that might follow a particular decision or action. The probability of these individual events is calculated and shown in parentheses. At the far right of the tree, the pay-off or the outcome for each branch will be calculated, taking into account the combination of an action or decision and its immediate consequences (Hill, et al., 1978; Hodgetts, 1979).

A Sample Decision Tree

As an illustration of how one might use a decision tree we can use the decision faced by an 87-year-old invalid widow. Symptoms indicate that she may have an inoperable dormant tumor but it cannot be diagnosed for certain. Ignore the possible tests that you know might be done and accept this hypothetical situation in which there is a 50/50 chance that the original problem, an inoperable dormant tumor, actually exists. The decision is whether or not to prescribe medication to prevent a reactivation of the suspected malignant growth. The medication being considered is effective but has some side effects, which may be minor or serious.

To arrange these possibilities in a decision tree, we start with our initial decision and draw our branches to the right, taking each event in turn. The final arrangement is shown in Figure 10.1.

The decision tree in Figure 10.1 is not complete. There are several possibilities not included, but the two basic alternatives illustrate the method. To complete the decision tree we must add two elements, an assigned value for each outcome and a probability estimate for each event. Then we will be ready to analyze the tree and come to a decision.

Completion of the Decision Tree

Assigning a value to each potential outcome is done on the far right side of the tree. The outcome of a course of action with its series of chance events that result in no further problems can be assigned a value of zero. Any outcome that does not result in this ideal outcome would merit a larger or smaller negative value, depending on how closely the outcome approximates the ideal of no further problem. In this case, if the outcome of a decision is a minor complication from the medication, the value might be set at -1. If the complications are more serious, a value of -2 might be appropriate. If the original serious problem recurs, the outcome could have a value of -3. If the original problem recurs and is complicated by side effects of the medication, we might assign a -4 if side effects are minor and a -5 if they are more serious. The assigned values for each outcome are placed in a circle after the appropriate outcome (Fig. 10.2).

Next we need to estimate the probability of as many events as we can in this tree. To simplify our illustration we can assume that medical research has already been done and we have good statistics to use in filling in the probabilities for each chance event. Table 10.1 lists these probabilities. All of these probabilities have been entered in parentheses in Figure 10.2. If solid probability figures are not available one can estimate the probabilities.

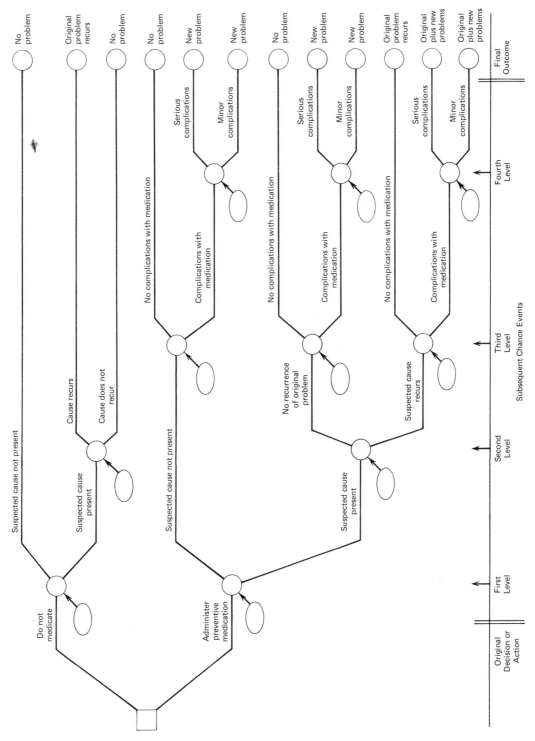

FIGURE 10.1 *Decision tree showing the original two decisions or actions considered, their possible or likely consequences (chance events), and final outcomes.*

TABLE 10.1   Chance Events and Their Probabilities

Event	Probability (%)	Event	Probability (%)
Tumor is present	50	Tumor is absent	50
Tumor reactivates	35	Tumor remains dormant	65
Medication causes side effects	90	Medication causes no side effects	10
Side effects are major	20	Side effects are minor	80

This step completes construction of our decision tree. Learning to use this diagram is our next task.

Analyzing the Decision Tree and Coming to a Decision

Now we can analyze our statistics to arrive at the optimal decision. We do this by "rolling back" our tree from right to left. Start at the far right bottom in Figure 10.2 with the assigned value for the last outcome, -4. Multiply this figure by the probability of that outcome, 80%: $-4 \times 0.8 = -3.2$. Move to the next line up and multiply the -5 outcome by the 20% probability: $-5 \times 0.2 = -1.0$. Add these two subtotals and you have the *calculated value* for the node leading to these two outcomes: $-3.2 + -1.0 = -4.2$. This calculated value is entered in a circle with an arrow pointing to the node (Fig. 10.3).

The next outcome, moving up the branches on the far right, can be ignored for the moment because it comes from a node on the third level rather than from the fourth level. We will work with it when we roll back to the third level. The next pair of outcomes from a fourth level node gives us the following calculations: $(-1.0 \times 0.80) + (-2 \times 0.20) = -1.2$.

The next outcome stems from the third level and is also ignored for the moment. The next set of calculations is a repeat of the second calculations, yielding a value of -1.2. This completes all the calculated values for the fourth level.

Rolling back to the third level and the bottom node, the figures are $(-4.2 \times 0.9) + (-3 \times 0.1) = -4.08$.

The calculated value for the next node up on the third level is $(-1.2 \times 0.10) + (0 \times 0.1) = -1.08$.

The last calculated value for the third level is a repeat of the one just done: -1.08.

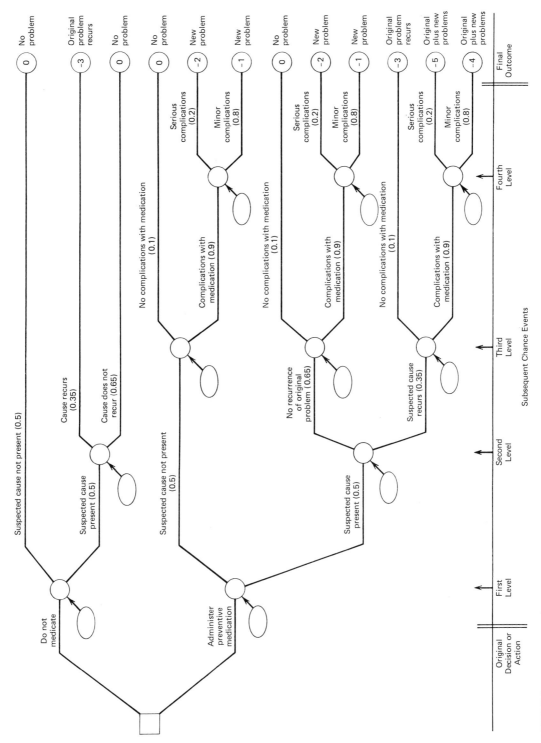

FIGURE 10.2 *Same decision tree shown in Figure 10.1, with assigned values listed for each final outcome on the far right and with probability estimates given in parentheses for each chance event.*

123

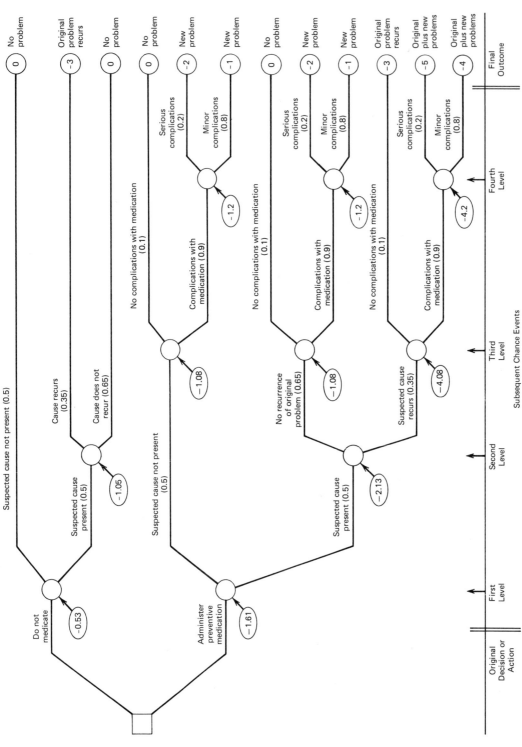

FIGURE 10.3 Completed version of Figure 10.1 decision tree. Calculated values have been worked out for each event node and entered in the oblong boxes with arrow pointing to the event node.

Calculated values for the two nodes on the second level are as follows:
$$(-4.08 \times 0.35) + (-1.08 \times 0.65) = -2.13$$
$$(-3 \times 0.35) + (0 \times 0.65) = -1.05$$
Calculated values for the final nodes, on the first level, are as follows:
$$(-2.13 \times 0.5) + (-1.08 \times 0.5) = -1.61$$
$$(-1.05 \times 0.5) + (0 \times 0.5) = -0.53$$
The optimal decision revealed by this decision tree is the alternative action with the lowest first level calculated value, in this case a value of -0.53 compared with a calculated value of -1.61. The decision is not to give the preventive medication.

Using the Decision Tree With Your Case Study

Having calculated the optimal ethical decision using the decision tree, you can work through a case of your own or a case assigned to you in class by using the exercise in Part Two.

REFERENCES AND FURTHER READINGS

Hill, P., et al. *Making Decisions: A Multidisciplinary Introduction*. Reading, MA: Addison-Wesley, 1978, pp. 152–176.

Hodgetts, R. *Management Theory, Process, and Practice*. Philadelphia: W.B. Saunders, 1979, pp. 198–202. Introductory texts on business management always contain good illustrations of decision trees and their applications.

11 THE DECISION MATRIX TECHNIQUE

CHAPTER 11

THE DECISION MATRIX TECHNIQUE

Most of the situations and ethical decisions encountered in the delivery of health care present several possible options. A *decision matrix* is one of the more structured and, at the same time, more useful ways of facilitating the choice of alternative that best serves the interests of the patient (Hill et al., 1978, Chap. 8). In some disciplines, such as futures studies, this technique is known as a *cross-matrix impact analysis*. Whatever name we give the technique, its most important characteristic is that its efficiency and usefulness increase when we have more alternatives from which to choose.

You can use the decision matrix to select which college major is best for you, which make of automobile to buy, or which alternative will assure the best and most ethically responsible health care for everyone affected in a situation. This approach to decision making is similar in many respects to the decision balance sheet (Chapter 9) and the decision tree (Chapter 10). However, because it is more mathematically structured, failure to identify *all* the relevant options will definitely distort your calculations and outcome. The matrix technique forces you into a mathematical analysis of each alternative in light of specific criteria you select and the varying weights you give these criteria. Attention to detail is vital.

CASE STUDY: LAW ON VITAL ORGAN BANK STIRS FRENCH CONTROVERSY

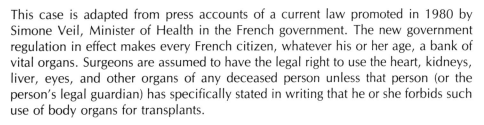

This case is adapted from press accounts of a current law promoted in 1980 by Simone Veil, Minister of Health in the French government. The new government regulation in effect makes every French citizen, whatever his or her age, a bank of vital organs. Surgeons are assumed to have the legal right to use the heart, kidneys, liver, eyes, and other organs of any deceased person unless that person (or the person's legal guardian) has specifically stated in writing that he or she forbids such use of body organs for transplants.

After both chambers of the French Parliament passed the bill in 1980, various groups and individuals began questioning the implications of the law. A new organization, the National Patients' Association, was formed to protest the law. The members of the group distributed "life passport" cards on the street and in public places in hope that everyone subject to the law would carry a signed statement accepting or refusing the use of his or her organs for transplant.

One of the most vocal opponents of the law was the conservative Parisian daily newspaper, *Le Figaro,* which claimed that the law is "revolutionary" and a deadly blow to "the religious spirit that commands respect for the dead."

The law requires every hospital to have a special register that patients or their families can sign to indicate their unwillingness to allow transplants. Any patient who does not sign the register is assumed to be agreeable to donating organs. One of the strongest objections to the bill is that most people will not bother to register when they are healthy. When they are injured or sick, they and their families are often not in a condition to make the decision. On the other side, physicians argue that the needs of the living must take precedence. In the year before the law went into effect over 1,000 cornea and over 800 kidney transplants were performed in France. The need for organs suitable for transplant is growing by at least 50% each year.

The new law requires prior authorization from parents or guardians for minors and the mentally retarded, and prohibits transplants in cases where autopsies are required to document the cause of death.

The law also redefines the medicolegal concept of death in terms laid down by the National Academy of Medicine and the National Council of the Order of Physicians. Cerebral death, the overriding factor, must be established by clinical observation by two physicians, one of them of senior rank at the hospital, and by tests, including an electroencephalogram.

Some interesting new views and interpretations have been prompted by the new law. Author Christiane Rochefort, for instance, sees the new law as a simple, logical extension of the expanding needs for raw materials we are witnessing in all industries. Organ transplantation is an expanding industry and we have to make provisions for its basic need for essential raw materials, human organs.

Phase One

Our first step in using a decision matrix is to identify all the alternatives we find ethically acceptable in this case. Since we are concerned in this worktext with approaches and decision-making processes rather than with conclusions, our sample case is simplified by using only three alternatives. If we were seriously concerned about the outcome, we would identify all possible alternatives and select several of the more important ones for analysis in our matrix instead of working with only the three below. Remember that the efficiency of the decision matrix increases in proportion to the number of alternatives you analyze.

1. The new law should remain in effect with interested groups such as the National Patients' Association free to promote life passports or other means of protecting those who oppose being organ donors.

2. The new law should be abolished and organ transplants done only when next of kin or the potential donor authorizes it. The government should not be involved in any way in promoting organ transplants.

3. The new law should be abolished and replaced with a uniform anatomical gift act similar to that adopted by several states in the United States. The Uniform Anatomical Gift Act allows a person to designate all or any body organs or parts for the purpose of transplantation, therapy, medical research, or education upon his or her death. A person interested in being a donor completes a card and signs it. When carried on one's person or attached to a driver's license, the card is legal authority for the use of body parts or organs indicated.

Phase Two

Our second step in the decision matrix process is to decide which criteria to use in evaluating our three alternatives. Since our objective is to identify the most ethical alternatives, we can begin with the six ethical principles we discussed in Chapter 3. When values and guidelines derived from these six principles are applied to our three alternatives, we can discover which values are promoted or harmed by each of the alternatives. Along with these ethical criteria, we may also want to include some economic, political, legal, or psychological criteria that have little or no moral content. As in our general and ethical weighting of consequences in the alternatives balance sheet (Chapter 9), nonethical values may not be primary in our decision, although they are worth considering.

In Chapter 3 we established six basic general ethical principles:

1. Personal autonomy

2. Veracity, or truth telling

3. Nonmaleficence, or not doing harm

4. Beneficence, or contributing to the good and welfare of others

5. Confidentiality

6. Justice, or equals should be treated equally and unequals should be treated unequally

Four of these principles apply to our sample case: personal autonomy, non-maleficence, beneficence, and justice.

Any two persons applying these four ethical principles to our case will inevitably come to different conclusions. While we might all agree on the general ethical principles, it is a different matter when we try to apply these to the specific issues of our sample case, or to those of any other case. As you may recall from the example in Chapter 3 about the ethics of testing measles vaccine on children, Ramsey and McCormick both agreed on the principles of justice and autonomy. Yet Ramsey felt that such nontherapeutic experimentation is not ethical; even though it benefits others and posed little risk to the children, it should be freely consented to as a charitable act not required by justice. For Ramsey, the principle of autonomy is more applicable to this case than the principle of justice. McCormick, on the other hand, saw such experimentation as coming under the principle of justice, which requires that everyone contribute to the welfare of fellow humans. If the parents consent, if there is minimal risk, and if it is medically sound, McCormick felt that the experimentation would be ethical. For McCormick, the moral obligation of justice outweighs the right to autonomy in this case.

To establish the specific criteria for our decision matrix, we have to deal with each of the four principles separately. Certain assumptions will be made, with which you may or may not agree. (You may suggest other values that you find more important, although we are interested here more in the method than in the outcome.) When you do your own matrix, you will naturally derive your own ethical values from the same six moral principles in keeping with your own sensitivity and conscience.

DERIVING VALUES FROM ETHICAL PRINCIPLES

Taking the first of our four ethical principles, autonomy, we need to explore specific values or criteria in this principle that apply to our case.

Under the principle of autonomy we might identify the following two guidelines or values as criteria. (1) A person should have total control over his or her own body, while alive. If someone wants to donate an organ for transplant while alive, he or she should be free to do so. (2) A person should have control over the disposition of his or her corpse after death. If one wants to make his or her organs available for transplant after death, he or she should be free to make this desire known in a "living will" or some other legal document.

TABLE 11.1   Criteria Derived from Ethical Principles Applicable to the Sample Case

Value	Order	Weighting Factor
(1) A person should have total control over his or her own body while alive.	7	$7 \div 28 = 0.26$
(3) We should never needlessly inflict harm on another human.	6	$6 \div 28 = 0.21$
(5) We should treat others as we would like them to treat us.	5	$5 \div 28 = 0.18$
(7) We should promote equitable distribution of rare resources such as organs for transplant.	4	$4 \div 28 = 0.14$
(4) Wherever possible, we should try to prevent harm befalling another human.	3	$3 \div 28 = 0.10$
(6) Each of us bears a responsibility to help other humans when there is minimal risk, harm, or inconvenience to us.	2	$2 \div 28 = 0.07$
(2) A person should have control over disposition of his or her corpse after death.	1	$1 \div 28 = 0.04$
TOTAL	28	$28 \div 28 = 1.0$

Under our second ethical principle, nonmaleficence, we might include two values as applicable criteria: (3) we should never needlessly inflict harm on another human; and (4) wherever possible we should try to prevent harm befalling another human.

The principle of beneficence is similar to the "golden rule": (5) we should treat others as we would like to be treated.

Following McCormick's analysis of the principle of justice, we reach this conclusion: (6) each of us bears a responsibility to help other human beings when there is minimal or no risk, harm, or inconvenience to us. At the same time we might include another value here: (7) we should promote the equitable distribution of rare resources (organs for transplant).

Our next task is to arrange these seven values or criteria in order of their importance to us (Table 11.1). In the following sample ranking, ignore for the moment the calculations on the right side of the table.

To give each of these seven values a weighting factor we simply assign our most important criteria a 7 and the least important criteria a 1. These figures, listed in the order column of our table, are added together. Each order figure is then divided by the sum, 28, to give us a weighting factor for each criteria. These calculations are already shown in Table 11.1.

However, if you look at our sample list of criteria again, you may decide that two or more of the ethical values have about the same importance. In this case, you should give them the same score. You might also decide that you could use a scale slightly larger than seven to spread out the criteria and better indicate their relative importance and relation to each other. In Table 11.2 this is done as an example, with 8 being the highest order number.

Control of one's body while alive still has first priority in this revised list, but the next three values of not inflicting harm, "doing unto others," and equitable distribution have been clustered together with an order weight of 5. The next two values are also linked together but with a smaller weight. The last value is of minimal concern so it remains at the bottom with a weight of only 1. No matter how these values are arranged or what weight you give each one, the process is the same: order divided by total equals the weighting factor.

At this point we could continue to Phase Three and construct our decision matrix chart. However, we have not included any nonmoral consequences or values in our ranking. As an example we might want to include in our table

TABLE 11.2   Revised Order Scale and Clustering of Values to Better Indicate Importance of Criteria

Value	Order	Weighting Factor
(1) A person should have total control over his or her own body while alive.	8	$8 \div 32 = 0.25$
(3) We should never needlessly inflict harm on another human.	5	$5 \div 32 = 0.15$
(5) We should treat others as we would like them to treat us.	5	$5 \div 32 = 0.15$
(7) We should promote equitable distribution of rare resources such as organs for transplant.	5	$5 \div 32 = 0.15$
(4) Wherever possible, we should try to prevent harm befalling another human.	4	$4 \div 32 = 0.13$
(6) Each of us bears a responsibility to help other humans when there is minimal risk, harm, or inconvenience to us.	4	$4 \div 32 = 0.13$
(2) A person should have control over disposition of his or her corpse after death.	1	$1 \div 32 = 0.04$
TOTAL	32	$32 \div 32 = 1.0$

TABLE 11.3   Third Revision Incorporating Predominantly Nonmoral Criteria or Objectives

Value	Order	Weighting Factor
Total control over body while alive	8	$8 \div 37 = 0.22$
Not inflicting harm needlessly	5	$5 \div 37 = 0.135$
Doing unto others as you would have them do unto you	5	$5 \div 37 = 0.135$
Equitable distribution of rare organs	5	$5 \div 37 = 0.135$
Preventing harm to others when possible	4	$4 \div 37 = 0.108$
Duty as neighbor's keeper	4	$4 \div 37 = 0.108$
Advancing medical knowledge	3	$3 \div 37 = 0.08$
Saving lives of "valuable" persons	2	$2 \div 37 = 0.054$
Disposition of one's corpse	1	$1 \div 37 = 0.27$
TOTAL	37	$37 \div 37 = 1.0$

some criteria or objectives with very little if any moral content. Two examples might be advancing medical knowledge and increased opportunity to save the lives of socially valuable persons. Advancing medical knowledge might carry more weight than the sanctity and autonomy of the human corpse, so an order of 3 might be appropriate. Extending the lives of socially important persons such as Mother Theresa, Beethoven, and the like might deserve a 2. Again, our table can be revised (Table 11.3).

Now we can proceed to Phase Three and incorporate these values in the decision matrix chart.

Phase Three

In constructing a decision matrix, list your alternatives down the left side of the chart (Fig. 11.1). Across the top of the chart list your selection criteria or values, both moral and nonmoral, starting with the highest value on the left and ending with the lowest value on the far right. Insert the final weighting factor for each criteria or value from Table 11.3.

Weighting factors ↓ / Selection values → \ Alternatives	Total control while alive	Don't harm needy or donors	Do unto others	Equitable distribution	Prevent harm to others	Neighbor's keeper	Advance medical knowledge	Save valuable lives	Disposition of dead body	SUM
	.22	.135	.135	.135	.108	.108	.08	.054	.027	1.0
Keep new law	10	10	10	10	8	8	3	3	0	
Abolish new law	10	2	0	0	10	1	0	0	10	
Abolish law; pass UAGA	10	9	8	9	10	3	3	3	10	

FIGURE 11.1   *Sample decision matrix with four sets of data entered to illustrate early stages of this technique: (1) alternatives, (2) selection values for the alternatives, (3) weighting factors, and (4) assigned rating factors.*

(Format from Hill, P., et al. *Making Decisions: A Multidisciplinary Introduction*. Reading, MA: Addison-Wesley, 1978, pp. 124–125. Reprinted with permission.)

Phase Four

The next task is to rate each of the alternatives, in this case only three, on a scale of 10 (highest) to 1 (lowest) to indicate the extent to which that alternative accomplishes or promotes a particular criterion or objective. This number is called a *rating factor* (RF).

All three alternatives give people total control over their bodies while alive, so each is given an RF value of 10. For our second criteria of not inflicting harm needlessly, option one deserves an RF value of 10. The second alternative of abolishing the donor law would needlessly harm many potential recipients of organ transplants, and thus perhaps deserves an RF of 2. The third alternative might be given an RF of 8 because it might still result in some shortage of organs for transplant. If you needed an organ transplant and this law would provide it, you would be concerned about the third objective or criterion; you might assign keeping the law an RF of 10, abolishing the law an RF of 0, and replacement of the law with a uniform anatomical gift act an RF of 8. The rest of Figure 11.1 has been completed to this point, one item at a time, criterion by criterion.

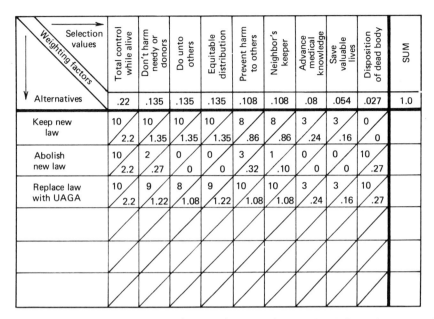

Weighting factors — Selection values / Alternatives	Total control while alive	Don't harm needy or donors	Do unto others	Equitable distribution	Prevent harm to others	Neighbor's keeper	Advance medical knowledge	Save valuable lives	Disposition of dead body	SUM
	.22	.135	.135	.135	.108	.108	.08	.054	.027	1.0
Keep new law	10 / 2.2	10 / 1.35	10 / 1.35	10 / 1.35	8 / .86	8 / .86	3 / .24	3 / .16	0 / 0	
Abolish new law	10 / 2.2	2 / .27	0 / 0	0 / 0	3 / .32	1 / .10	0 / 0	0 / 0	10 / .27	
Replace law with UAGA	10 / 2.2	9 / 1.22	8 / 1.08	9 / 1.22	10 / 1.08	10 / 1.08	3 / .24	3 / .16	10 / .27	

FIGURE 11.2 *Decision matrix form with spaces for entering information on products obtained from multiplying each combination of rating factor and weighting factor. These products should be entered in the appropriate lower half of each box.*

(Format from Hill, P., et al. *Making Decisions: A Multidisciplinary Introduction.* Reading, MA: Addison-Wesley, 1978, pp. 124–125. Reprinted with permission.)

Phase Five

Completing the decision matrix now requires only some simple mathematics with a calculator. Deal with each square separately. Multiply the appropriate weighting factor from the top of the column by the rating factor in the upper half of the square. Enter the product in the lower half of that square. Repeat this simple multiplication with each box until you have filled in the lower half of all the boxes in Figure 11.2.

Next, add up all the products in the *lower half* of the squares *across from the first alternative.* Enter this total in the box at the far right end of the line, under *sum.* Repeat this addition for the second and third alternatives (Fig. 11.3).

Finally, check the sums at the far right. The alternative with the highest sum has the *highest confidence level* and is the most ethical alternative. Now it is obvious why we stressed the need for serious and careful thought about selecting and weighting your criteria or objectives. To obtain valid results with the decision matrix, you must be very thorough and conscientious in determining which ethical principles, guidelines, and objectives are involved in your

Weighting factors / Selection values / Alternatives	Total control while alive	Don't harm needy or donors	Do unto others	Equitable distribution	Prevent harm to others	Neighbor's keeper	Advance medical knowledge	Save valuable lives	Disposition of dead body	SUM
	.22	.135	.135	.135	.108	.108	.08	.054	.027	1.0
Keep new law	10 / 2.2	10 / 1.35	10 / 1.35	10 / 1.35	8 / .86	8 / .86	3 / .24	3 / .16	0 / 0	8.37
Abolish new law	10 / 2.2	2 / .27	0 / 0	0 / 0	3 / .32	1 / .10	0 / 0	0 / 0	10 / .27	3.16
Replace new law with UAGA	10 / 2.2	9 / 1.22	8 / 1.08	9 / 1.22	10 / 1.08	10 / 1.08	3 / .24	3 / .16	10 / .27	8.55

FIGURE 11.3   *Completed sample of a decision matrix with the final stage sums entered on the far right.*

(Format from Hill, P., et al. *Making Decisions: A Multidisciplinary Introduction.* Reading, MA: Addison-Wesley, 1978, pp. 124–125. Reprinted with permission.)

case; in listing your alternatives; and in assigning the weighting and rating factors. If these early steps are not carefully executed, the results of the exercise will be misleading.

Applying the Decision Matrix to Your Case Study

To use the decision matrix exercise in Part Two, you may want a calculator to avoid making tedious calculations. Use a case of your own choice or one assigned to you in class. Remember that the early steps are vital to the success of your effort. Shading has been added to the matrix charts as a guide to filling in the appropriate boxes in each step.

REFERENCES AND FURTHER READINGS

Barry, V. *Moral Aspects of Health Care.* Belmont, CA: Wadsworth, 1982, pp. 480–483.

Beauchamp, T.L., & Childress, J.F. *Principles of Biomedical Ethics.* New York: Oxford University Press, 1979, pp. 231 233.

Davis, A.J., & Aroskar, M.A. *Ethical Dilemmas and Nursing Practice.* New York: Appleton-Century-Crofts, 1978, pp. 193–194.

Easton, A. *Decision Making: A Short Course in Problem Solving for Professionals,* Part 4, Step 5: Predict and quantify outcomes of alternatives on all criteria; Part 5, Steps 6 and 7: Translate outcome scores into value scores and weight criteria; and Part VI, Step 8: Select a rule and compute the best alternative. New York: John Wiley & Sons, 1976.

Fromer, M.J. *Ethical Issues in Health Care.* St. Louis: C.V. Mosby, 1981, pp. 341–369.

Gaylin, W. "Harvesting the dead." In Shannon, T.A., ed. *Bioethics: Basic Writings.* New York: Paulist Press, 1981, pp. 517–528.

Hill, P., et al. *Making Decisions: A Multidisciplinary Introduction.* Reading, MA: Addison-Wesley, 1978, pp. 120–127. The main structure of this chapter exercise is drawn from the explanation given in Hill.

McConnell, T.C. *Moral Issues in Health Care: An Introduction to Medical Ethics.* Monterey, CA: Wadsworth Health Sciences, 1982, pp. 235–249.

Munson, R., ed. *Intervention and Reflection: Basic Issues in Medical Ethics,* 2nd ed. Belmont, CA: Wadsworth, 1979, pp. 487–516.

CHAPTER 12

A TECHNIQUE FOR COPING WITH THE LEAST DESIRABLE OPTION

As part of a health care team, it is likely that you will encounter a situation in which the option to which you are most opposed is selected for implementation. It may be the decision of the physician in charge or of an ethics committee. If your ethical conflict is serious enough, you may ask to be excused from the case, but it may also be difficult, if not impossible, to withdraw because of your position. Or, you may decide that by remaining a part of the health care team, you can do something to alleviate the harmful consequences you anticipate. Trying to reduce the harmful consequences of a decision you have no authority to change may be an ethical alternative when what you see as the most ethical option is ignored. In trying to reduce the harmful consequences you can achieve at least some of your ethical goals.

Finding ways of coping with the ethically least desirable option is the objective of this exercise.* Our sample case is an unusual one that could only exist because of our recent advances in genetics, fetal monitoring, immunology, and aerospace technology. The case was the subject of a melodramatic television movie of the late 1970s, in which John Travolta played the lead as the "Bubble Boy."

CASE STUDY: DAVID, THE "BUBBLE BOY"

In 1982 David celebrated his eleventh birthday. He has had an unusual childhood. Having been born with severe combined immunodeficiency disease (SCID), David is its longest surviving sufferer. The disease leaves David with no functioning B or T cells, two of the vital components of the body's immune system. These cells,

---

*The format for this exercise is adapted from "A Comprehensive Study of the Ethical, Legal, and Social Implications for Advances in Biomedical and Behavioral Research and Technology," a nationwide survey of experts and lay persons conducted by Policy Research Inc., 2500 North Charles St., Baltimore, MD 21218, and the Center for Technology Assessment, New Jersey Institute of Technology, 323 High Street, Newark, NJ 07102.

derived from bone marrow, combat viral and bacterial infections. Without them, the slightest common bacterial or viral contact could prove lethal to David.

Because his family and physicians were prepared, David survived the transition from a safe uterine environment to this microorganism-packed world. Three years before, David's mother had had a son who had died within a few days of birth. The postmortem revealed a hereditary, sex-linked recessive form of SCID. This meant that any boy the couple might have would have a 50/50 chance of immuno-deficiency; any girls would be free of the gene or would be normal carriers like their mother. When the wife became pregnant a second time, amniocentesis was performed. The second child, a girl, posed no problem. During the third pregnancy, amniocentesis revealed a boy with SCID, yet the couple decided against an early abortion. As soon as David was delivered by Ceasarean section he was placed in a sterile incubator. For the past 11 years, David has never been outside of some form of sterile isolation environment.

Until November 1977, David was limited to a transparent plastic three-room, 6-foot-high sterile home in the living room of his parent's house near Houston, Texas. Then, through space technology, David received from NASA a $20,000 miniature space suit attached by a 10-foot umbilical cord to a life-support unit on wheels. For the first time, David left his three-room plastic home and walked around the front yard. At first David was afraid of tripping, but after his first tumble, he got up, laughed, and walked again. He quickly became comfortable with his new suit. However, he has only one outing a month because of the need for constant mon-itoring by specially trained personnel.

David has given his parents one real scare in all his years at home in the "bubble." He swallowed a coin, which lodged in his throat. Fortunately, surgery was avoided by using a fiberoptic bronchoscope to remove the coin with forceps.

Although David's only contact with other people is through the rubber gloves in the portholes of his plastic home, pediatricians and child psychiatrists who have worked with David say he has no serious psychological problems. He has never been touched directly, never cuddled against another person's body, never smelled another's breath. Yet the problems that we would expect from this deprivation of nurturance, especially in the early years, seem simply not to have occurred with David.

How many more years David will have to remain in his sterile environment is not known. Doctors have ruled out the usual thymosin treatment to stimulate his immune system. A search of thousands of would-be bone marrow donors has not yet turned up a suitable match. Normal bone marrow would produce the needed B and T cells, but unless the transplanted marrow is an exact immunologic match of the recipient's marrow, the donor immune cells will attack and destroy the re-cipient's cells. In late 1982 a new treatment was announced that might help David. Donor bone marrow is treated with monoclonal antibodies designed to attack ma-ture T cells in the marrow and with protein complement that helps control the body's immune system. The T cells are the ones that cause mismatched marrow to produce graft-versus-host rejection. With 99% of the culprit T cells removed, the donor marrow has time, with subsequent treatment, to adjust to its new environment without rejecting it. This new technique may be David's best hope of living a normal life. Until then, he continues his life in a sterile environment.

Four Alternatives for This Case

Four alternatives might be suggested as ways of handling similar situations in which couples known to be at risk for passing on SCID decide to try to have children despite the odds. These alternatives would not affect infants born with SCID to couples who had no suspicion of their being at risk.

1. *Refusal of medical support.* Any couple known to be at risk for bearing children with SCID should be warned that physicians and hospitals cannot provide the very expensive and extraordinary health care a newborn with SCID needs. If the couple decides to continue the pregnancy despite the risk, even after amniocentesis proves that the fetus suffers from SCID, then they will have to pay for the treatment. If they cannot pay, they will have to accept the natural outcome and consequences of their decision.

2. *Refusal of government support.* The federal and state government agencies that support these physicians and hospitals should halt funds for SCID research and divert the money saved to other health care programs that benefit many more people.

3. *No restrictions or limitations.* Couples known to be at risk for bearing children with SCID should have no restrictions placed on their right to have as many children as they desire. Physicians and society should respect their wishes and provide whatever medical care is needed.

4. *Limitation of childbirth.* Couples known to be at risk for bearing children with SCID should be allowed to have more children if they wish. However, each subsequent pregnancy must be monitored. If amniocentesis shows that the fetus has SCID, medical insurance should pay for an abortion. If the couple decides not to have an abortion, no extraordinary care should be paid for by medical insurance.

Which of these four alternatives is your *least* desirable option?

For our example we use the fourth option as our least desirable alternative and try to devise ways of coping with the negative consequences we might anticipate for this option.

Phase One

When working with our least desirable option—limiting childbearing for couples known to be at risk for bearing children with SCID—we need to identify the three most negative consequences of this ethically least desirable alternative. Since this alternative obviously affects the personal autonomy of such couples, the issue of pressured abortion, and the future of medical research on SCID, we might list the following as the three important negative consequences of this least desirable option:

1. This alternative would be a dangerous violation of the basic right of every individual to reproduce, which could easily be extended to other areas of genetic control and eugenic design.

2. Powerful and perhaps irresistible pressures would be brought to bear on couples opposed to abortion on religious grounds.

3. Such restrictions would severely hamper the efforts of medical science to advance its knowledge of the immune response and immunodeficiency diseases.

These three negative consequences more or less directly affect different parties, whom we should identify before giving some detail on the consequences. Among those who might be harmed in this or any other case are the following:

____ Ethnic or racial minorities

____ Illegal aliens

____ People in other countries

____ Urban Americans

____ Rural Americans

____ Low-income persons

____ Middle-income persons

____ Wealthy persons

____ Children under 18

____ Adults 18 to 35

____ Adults 36 to 60

____ Adults over 60

____ College-educated persons

____ High school graduates

____ Persons with elementary school education only

____ Healthy persons

____ Acutely ill persons

____ Chronically ill persons

____ Institutionalized persons

____ Prison inmates

____ Unemployed welfare recipients

____ Biomedical researchers

____ Private industry

—— Insurance companies

—— Pharmaceutical companies

—— Government

—— Health care professionals

—— Other (specify)

Review this list and mark those parties most likely to be harmed by the three negative consequences identified above. Then continue with Phase Two.

Phase Two

In this section we examine each of the three negative consequences before we try to devise ways to ameliorate the situation.

FIRST NEGATIVE CONSEQUENCE

The first negative consequence is a dangerous violation of the basic right of every adult to bear children, and could easily be extended to endorse genetic control and eugenic design. Among the parties listed above who might suffer most from this first negative consequences are:

People with a limited education who would find it difficult to understand the basic hereditary principles and genetic risks.

Ethnic or racial minorities in whom other serious hereditary diseases are more common than in the population as a whole. Discrimination could easily follow this alternative.

The poor and middle-income couples who cannot afford special treatment.

With these affected parties in mind, we can explain some of the details of our briefly stated consequence. Analyzing this consequence, we might break it up into several areas of concern, as follows:

1. Our civil and religious traditions have always assumed that every adult has an inalienable right to reproduce. This right would be denied to some people not because of anything they did, but because of their heredity.

2. This alternative would set a dangerous precedent for extending regulations prohibiting reproduction to couples at risk for having children with cystic fibrosis, hemophilia, Tay-Sachs disease, Huntington's disease, and others.

3. People with only an elementary education might find it difficult to understand the genetic principles and the concept of risk for a future child.

4. The rich might ignore the ban, thereby creating discrimination based on wealth—if you can pay, your child lives; if you cannot pay, your child dies.

5. Once the door is opened to this kind of restriction or limitation on who reproduces, it will be easy to approve genetic designing of future humans.

Can you think of some other points to include under an explanation of this consequence?

_____

_____

_____

_____

SECOND NEGATIVE CONSEQUENCE

Powerful and perhaps irresistible pressures will be brought to bear on couples who cannot accept abortion because of moral or religious reasons. Three parties would be very much affected by this second consequence:

Adult couples opposed to abortion

Newborn infants with SCID, who would be doomed to early death

Insurance companies, which will become moderators of social standards if they are allowed to pick and choose which hereditary diseases are acceptable or not acceptable for coverage under their policies.

Can you think of any one else who might be affected by this second negative consequence?

_____

_____

Elaborating on this second negative consequence, we might suggest the following:

1. A human life is sacred. Once a fetus enters this world its life deserves protection. The newborn is helpless and dependent. To allow it to die as punishment for a parental decision is unjust.

2. No matter how indirect the pressure, this alternative is an infringement on the religious beliefs of those who believe the fetus is endowed with human rights. Through private business and insurance companies, government will be infringing on constitutional rights and setting a dangerous legal precedent.

3. If this policy were instituted, insurance companies and private health maintenance organizations could exercise considerable authority in deciding who should and should not reproduce.

Are there any other details you would want to include under this second consequence?

_____

_____

_____

_____

_____

THIRD NEGATIVE CONSEQUENCE

The parties most affected by the third negative consequence of our least desirable alternative, hindering medical research, would be the following:

- Medical researchers

- The chronically ill with autoimmune diseases

- Children with immune disease problems

We might raise some of the following points to explain this negative consequence:

1. Obviously, if couples are severely discouraged from having children when there is a risk of SCID, far fewer infants will be born with the disease. With research on SCID severely cut back, many people who develop immune deficiencies or autoimmune diseases later in life will not benefit from insights that might have been gained from research on neonatal SCID and its possible control or cure. Arthritic persons might be the main victims of the cut-back.

2. Those infants who are accidentally born with SCID will suffer since there will be even less incentive to research their problem. We have enough orphan diseases without adding to the list.

3. If we are going to deny treatment to SCID children born to parents at risk, some might urge that it would be more humane to hasten their inevitable death by legalizing mercy killing under such special circumstances.

Can you add any other details or comments to this third negative consequence?

_____

_____

_____

_____

Phase Three

With these insights into the types of negative consequences we can expect from our least desirable alternative, we now focus in on the objective of this exercise: How can we reduce the harm created by this least desirable option? What might we do to ameliorate the situation when we decide to remain part of the group involved in the case or when the decision is unalterable?

As an example, suggestions for reducing the harmful effects of our third negative consequence, hindering medical research, might include the following:

1. Funds previously devoted to SCID research should be redirected to support research on other immunologic problems, including arthritis.

2. Biomedical researchers should be encouraged with grants to develop animal models of SCID research.

3. Efforts might be increased to develop a safe, accurate prenatal test that could diagnose SCID in the first trimester and thereby allow the parents to make an early decision on abortion.

You can probably think of other ways to reduce the harm of the third consequence. Use the space below to spell out your suggestions for reducing the harm of the *first two consequences.*

For the *first negative consequence,* what specific policies, laws, guidelines, regulations, or other steps can you recommend to limit the invasion of personal rights to an absolute minimum? How would you minimize the potential for genetic control and eugenic design by society, business, or government? If you cannot reduce the harm to an acceptable level, what can you do to compensate those who actually suffer harm from this consequence? A class or small group discussion of possible remedies often leads to unusual and creative solutions. State your ideas concisely in the space below.

_____

_____

_____

_____

_____

_____

_____

_____

_____

_____

_____

For the *second negative consequence,* answer the same questions posed above for the first negative consequence. State your ideas concisely in the space below.

_____

_____

_____

_____

_____

_____

_____

_____

_____

_____

_____

_____

_____

Applying This Exercise to Your Case Study

Having observed this technique in action, you should now be able to use it with your own case study or with a case study provided by your instructor. Work slowly; this is one of the more difficult of our decision-making exercises. It is not easy to think in negative terms, but this ability can be helpful in developing your decision-making skills. An exercise for this chapter can be found in Part Two of this worktext.

REFERENCES AND FURTHER READINGS

Davis, A.J., & Aroskar, M.A. *Ethical Dilemmas and Nursing Practice.* New York: Appleton-Century-Crofts, 1978, pp. 79–80, 116–129.

Havighurst, C.G. "Compensating persons injured in human experimentation." In Wertz, R.W., ed. *Readings on Ethical and Social Issues in Biomedicine.* Englewood Cliffs, NJ: Prentice-Hall, 1973, pp. 50–54.

Janis, I.L., & Mann, L. *Decision Making: A Psychological Analysis of Conflict, Choice and Commitment.* New York: Free Press, 1977, pp. 219–242, 243–278, 309–338.

McConnell, T.C. *Moral Issues in Health Care.* Monterey, CA: Wadsworth Health Sciences, 1982, pp. 116–154.

Munson, R., ed. *Intervention and Reflection: Basic Issues in Medical Ethics,* 2nd ed. Belmont, CA: Wadsworth, 1979, pp. 473–558.

Policy Research Incorporated and the Center for Technology Assessment, New Jersey Institute of Technology. *A Comprehensive Study of the Ethical, Legal, and Social Implications of Advances in Biomedical and Behavioral Research and Technology.* Baltimore: Policy Research Inc., 1975. The central exercise in this chapter is based on a polyevaluation instrument adapted from this nationwide study mandated by the National Commission for the Protection of Human Subjects of Biomedical and Behavioral Research.

Purtilo, R.B., & Cassel, C.K. *Ethical Dimensions in the Health Professions.* Philadelphia: W.B. Saunders, 1981, pp. 204–207.

NOTES

13 ASCERTAINING THE EFFECTS OF MOTIVATIONS ON DECISIONS

CHAPTER 13

ASCERTAINING THE EFFECTS OF MOTIVATIONS ON DECISIONS

Personal motives play a large role in the decisions of the people involved in a problem situation. What people say and their actions spring from motives that are often never articulated. In making decisions about ethical dilemmas in health care, how much weight should we give the various motives of others? How important are our own motives? How can these subtle motives be weighed? To what extent, if any, should they be considered in our decision-making process?

Chauncey Leake, considered by many to be the dean of medical ethics, has studied the variety of motives encountered in cases of organ transplants. "The recipient of a transplant," Leake notes, "is motivated by hedonism; he wants to continue to live and continue to get all the happiness he can. The donor may be motivated by an idealistic point of view, of being willing to sacrifice even something of himself for the recipient. The doctor does not think of this at all. All he is interested in is whether or not it works. My point is that in this situation there's a clash of three basic ethical principles" (American Medical News, 1972). How do we resolve a conflict like this among a hedonistic recipient, an altruistic donor, and a pragmatic physician? What weight do we give their conflicting motives?

Perhaps the situation would change significantly if Leake had pictured a quite different set of motives. The recipient might be willing to undergo the painful transplant out of concern for a dependent spouse or children rather than from a hedonistic desire to continue living at any cost. The donor might be a relative or friend more interested in gaining favor with the rich recipient in hopes of a healthy inheritance than in any altruistic concern. Physicians are often more altruistic than pragmatic, yet some have a hedonistic financial motive. Moreover, few of our motives are purely pragmatic, purely altruistic, or purely hedonistic. Most of them are a mixture of many interests combined in different proportions. Thus, answering the question of what importance we should give our motives and those of others in reaching ethical decisions about health care becomes a truly complex puzzle.

As an opening illustration of how motives can be a factor in making decisions, we might use a situation involving the patient's right to know the extent and nature of her condition and the ethical responsibility of others to inform and not to deceive the patient.

A 50-year-old woman complains that she has not been feeling well. She has lost weight without apparent reason and is complaining of abdominal pains and elimination problems. After several visits to her family physician, he recommends an abdominal x-ray examination. When this fails to reveal anything, she is given a complete gastrointestinal barium enema series, which reveals metastasized inoperable cancer. The prognosis is that she will live about 2 years. Her husband died of the same type of cancer 6 years ago.

Before informing the woman of her condition, the physician consults with the woman's only child, a nurse in the same hospital. The physician does not want to tell the woman that she has terminal cancer. His motive is to make her remaining time as normal as possible and to avoid the risk of her losing hope and dying prematurely. The daughter wants to inform her mother so that she does not have to carry the burden of knowledge alone. She worries about letting the information slip out or arousing her mother's suspicions.

The main ethical issue here is the principle of autonomy as it involves the mother's right to be informed about her condition, but the motives of the daughter and the physician do enter into the decision-making process. The physician could just as easily favor telling the mother because of her right to informed consent. The daughter could just as easily not want her mother told since there is nothing for which the woman needs to give informed consent. The daughter might also believe that her mother would become seriously depressed if told because of the husband's death from cancer.

When it comes to analyzing motives, we need to ask some important questions:

• To what extent do we take into consideration the motives of the different persons involved?

• How much weight do we, or should we, give these motives?

• Are there any situations in which the motives of one of the people in the situation might be the dominant element in deciding what is the most ethical action?

The Case of GG

Instead of using an everyday ethical situation from clinical practice, it might be more helpful to use instead a "mind-stretching" example. Walter Bornemeier (1966) has devised such a case in his account of "GG." Grandpa's Grandpa—GG to his friends and family—illustrates some of the issues raised by medical technology's growing ability to prolong life. What makes the case particularly useful for us are two characteristics: first, the account contains very little mention of motives; second, there is no mention of GG's personality and the relationships that bind him to his family. (This double deficiency reminds us of the importance of the "feminine" moral perspective examined by Gilligan in Chapter 2.)

Read the case slowly two or three times. As you read, look for any clues you can find to the possible motives of GG himself, his family, his physicians, and the 25-year-old great grandnephew who wrote this report.

CASE STUDY: GRANDPA'S GRANDPA: A SCENARIO FOR TOMORROW

Grandpa's Grandpa was scheduled to die tomorrow, but three members of the family said they positively couldn't get away for his funeral any time soon, so the demise of Grandpa's Grandpa was postponed again, giving him his sixth new lease on life.

He's a very old man now and a lot of grandpas have come and gone in our family in his time. That's why we call him GG for short, to tell him apart from the others.

GG died once, but at the time he was in the hospital having surgery for a hernia. When his failing heart stopped, they hooked him up to an artificial heart and restored his life. That was more than 50 years ago, when GG was about 75, and the doctors and nurses who performed that hook-up are now gone.

What with social security, medicare, and his annuity, GG has always had good care and has never really been an invalid. He has had a couple of leg fractures and an occasional bout of asthma or indigestion, but on the whole his health is good, considering his 125 years. He weighs only 90 pounds, so it doesn't cost much to keep him—two small meals a day and a bit of wine. He doesn't smoke and he sits so still that his clothing lasts for years, although it does get somewhat unfashionable.

The consensus seems to be that GG has a good disposition, otherwise the family would have let him die long ago—by just stealing the battery that runs his heart, for instance, or simply failing to replace it with a new one in June, causing a sure summer funeral.

About the time I was born, GG turned 100. That was the year when the family first decided that they should let GG pass away, a decision that, I understand, didn't come easily, but took the best part of an afternoon.

There was considerable opposition to letting GG die, mainly because he was not really in poor health for a man his age. But it was admitted that, although he had a heart in good working order, his brain was badly run down.

By a slim majority, GG was doomed. And then he was resurrected. Someone, who had reached a pretty high station in life by living by the rules, noted that a quorum was not present.

After that first meeting, the subject of GG's funeral didn't come up again for years, possibly because his health seemed to be getting even better, but probably because GG was becoming an asset while his heirs became fewer and fewer.

A small sum of money he had once invested had grown quite large over the years because he used little of the income and the rest just kept accumulating and compounding.

In the summer of his 110th year GG's fate was again discussed at a family meeting. No one mentioned it openly, I've been told, but everyone knew that if GG was allowed to die then, a no-good grandnephew would get a sizeable portion of the estate.

The vote was in favor of keeping GG with us, and a farsighted vote it was because the no-good heir passed on within the year.

With the no-gooder gone, there seemed little reason to prolong the old gentleman's life, so a special session was called. It was noted at the meeting that GG was becoming more forgetful and he sometimes refused to eat. But before the matter came to a vote, a couple of juniors enrolled in premed at one of the universities spoke up and said GG was becoming a valuable research specimen.

The logic of their arguments won over the rest of the family, and GG's funeral was put off for the third time.

At times though, it almost seemed as if the decision had not been a wise one. During the following winter, GG fell and broke his right leg. Later he fell and broke his left leg. Each time he was hospitalized for six weeks before returning home.

While in the hospital, the artificial prolongation of his life, which everybody agreed was really quite useless, became the subject of widespread debate among doctors, nurses, medical students, and orderlies.

Merely removing the stimulus to the artificial heart could not be considered murder, the argument went. After all, God had created GG with a heart and the heart was still present in the body. If the heart machine were turned off, then it was God's decision whether GG's human heart would function.

A meeting of the clan was called to discuss the wisdom of keeping GG alive, especially in the light of community pressure and gossip. But the family closed ranks—no outsiders were going to tell them what to do with their poor old Grandpa's Grandpa.

The fifth "make-the-decision" session, the first that I've attended, was rather serious because the nature of the problem had changed. A miraculous device had been invented which, if installed, would prolong GG's life indefinitely, possibly for hundreds of years.

Many problems had been created by the invention of that device, not the least of which was how to justify *not* using the machine. When Grandpa, at age 75, had become the recipient of an artificial heart, his existence had been presented to a future generation, to prolong or end as it thought best.

This new twist to the GG problem completely broke down the decision-making process. No decision was made—as I said before, three members of the family ended the discussion when they said they couldn't make it to a funeral, although we all knew that they really could.

So GG is 125 today, and I couldn't help thinking during the meeting . . .

The surgeon put a ticker in
To keep our Gramp alive.
But who will turn the gadget off
At a hundred twenty-five?
We often call a problem solved
Because it goes away.
And then we find to our chagrin
The same one's there next day.
But progress is our way of life,
So why should it seem strange.
If the questions must remain the same,
It's the answers that we'll change.

(Reprinted from Bornemeier, W. "Grandpa's Grandpa: A scenario for tomorrow," *Chicago Tribune Sunday Magazine,* June 26, 1966.)

Phase One

First we need to identify the main parties in our case. In the story of GG, we have four parties:

1. GG himself

2. GG's family

3. GG's doctors

4. The great grandnephew

Next, we need to select one option as a focus for the motives we attribute to these four parties. Among the options open to us in the story of GG, we could choose from the following:

1. Install the "miraculous device," the nuclear-powered artificial heart, and let GG live forever.

2. Continue replacing GG's battery, but do nothing else.

3. Let the battery run out in June and allow GG to die naturally.

There are, of course, other alternatives. For our purpose here, we can use the first option.

Phase Two

So far we have mentioned three different types of motives, *altruistic, pragmatic,* or *hedonistic,* but without defining these labels. For our purposes here, the following working definitions are useful:

• Altruistic: having an unselfish concern for others

• Pragmatic: practical, utilitarian, useful

• Hedonistic: concerned only with one's own pleasure and good

Labeling the few scraps of actual motives contained in Bornemeier's account of Grandpa's Grandpa is not too difficult. There are no clues to GG's thinking nor to the motives of the health professionals working with him. The family members seem to have mixed motives. At times they may be called pragmatic or hedonistic. For example, they will not let GG die if it will interrupt their vacations or if the "no-good grandnephew" will inherit the main part of the estate. The relatives who were medical students were pragmatic about GG being a "valuable research specimen." However, the motives that prompted a closing of ranks and the decision that no outsiders were to tell them what to do with GG do not seem to fit comfortably under any particular label. The great grandnephew who tells the story seems to be truly altruistic and concerned for GG, although he never describes his personal relationship with GG.

Since the story of GG provides very few actual motives, we can fill in the gaps with possible motives for the four parties. You can add your own insights to the sample motives suggested below.

THE CENTRAL PERSON IN THIS CASE (GRANDPA'S GRANDPA)

An altruistic motive for GG's desire to continue living might be that he wants to help solve some of the problems of aging by serving as a research subject. A hedonistic motive might be that *GG* enjoys living. A pragmatic motive might be that GG wants to avoid bickering and squabbling over his money, which his death would trigger.

Another motive that does not match these three labels might be that GG despises his relatives and doesn't want them to enjoy the money he worked so hard for.

What additional motives can you think of for GG? List them below.

_____

_____

_____

_____

_____

_____

THE SECOND PARTY OF PERSONS (GG'S FAMILY)

An altruistic motive for letting GG live might be that he should enjoy his money and life as long as he wants.

A hedonistic motive would be that GG's fantastic touch with the stock market could make them millionaires if he lives another 10 years.

Can you suggest some other motives for the family members?

_____

_____

_____

_____

_____

_____

THE THIRD PARTY (THE DOCTORS)

The doctors' altruistic motive might be that they want to help him to make life as comfortable and rich as they can for as long as GG wants to live. A hedonistic motive might be that they enjoy researching geriatric problems and GG is a perfect subject because he's much more cooperative than other patients and he pays their bills and supports their research.

A pragmatic motive would be that their success with this "machine" would make them sure candidates for a Nobel Prize in medicine.

What other motives can you suggest for GG's physicians? How would you label these motives?

_____

_____

_____

_____

_____

_____

THE FOURTH PARTY (THE GREAT GRANDNEPHEW)

An altruistic motive could be his love for and concern that GG have the fullest and most enjoyable life possible. A hedonistic motive might be the hope that he can get closer to GG and become his sole heir. A pragmatic motive might be that if GG becomes immortal, his favorite great grandnephew will benefit from the publicity, which would advance his career in public relations and advertising.

What other kinds of motives can you think of for the great grandnephew?

_____

_____

_____

_____

_____

_____

Phase Three

To fully appreciate the possible influence of motives on your decision you would need to analyze all possible motives for the other options in this case of GG the same way you analyzed the possible motives for the first option of giving GG immortality. This you can do on your own or in class with all the students contributing to a discussion on possible motives. For our illustration of this approach to decision making, we move directly to three important analytical questions.

First, how does your awareness of these motives affect or alter your selection of the most ethical option in this case? It might be that you are quite upset by any of the hedonistic, egotistic, or selfish motives. If you knew that GG wanted to live forever out of spite for his parasitic relatives, would you be inclined to put the research money into other "more worthy" projects that would benefit more people? In terms of distributive justice and doing the most good for the most people, would you then favor a preventive medicine project in the ghetto over spending money to keep GG alive for his selfish, egotistic reasons? Although GG has just as much right to live as anyone else, should limited money, limited skilled researchers, and limited equipment be used to benefit the most people?

Use the space below to express your own views on how awareness of these motives would affect your selection.

_____

_____

_____

_____

_____

_____

Second, what particular motive of one person in the case would lead you to consider changing your original decision on the most ethical option? Perhaps hedonistic or pragmatic reasons disturb you, particularly if the family, which appears to be making the decision, expresses them. If the family wants to keep GG alive only to avoid being disturbed on vacation or to make more money and if GG cannot express concern one way or the other, would you be inclined to let him die to avoid his being exploited?

Express your views on how a particular motive would lead you to change your original decision in the space below.

_____

_____

_____

_____

_____

_____

Third, in your list of actual and possible motives, can you find a combination of motives for two or three different persons which, when considered in tandem, might lead you to make a different decision?

One combination suggested by the analysis of the first option involves GG, the doctors, and GG's family. If GG only wants to live forever to spite his relatives, the doctors only want him alive so they can win the Nobel Prize, and the family only wants the fame of being descendants of the first immortal man, would it be ethical to invest more money and research in keeping him alive?

What combination of motives would you find unacceptable for the other two options of simply failing to replace the present battery or letting GG die in June?

_____

_____

_____

_____

_____

_____

Applying This Exercise to Your Case Study

You can now use the motivational analysis forms in the exercise in Part Two with a case of your own choice or with one assigned to you in class. Remember, to get a full picture of the impact of possible and real motives on your ethical decision, you should analyze the motives that could occur with each of the main options you identify. No matter how much or how little weight you give motives, they are factors you should consider. In the final analysis you may even decide to ignore motives in your decision, but you can only make that decision after you find out what the motives are and what weight they deserve.

REFERENCES AND FURTHER READINGS

Textbooks on biomedical ethics seldom mention the role of the participants' motives in resolving ethical dilemmas. General ethics texts are more likely to touch on the issue. Writings on the theory of just wars, particularly those by Paul Ramsey and Robert Tucker, frequently deal with the motive test and the question of intention. Writings in moral philosophy dealing with conscience often explore content and procedures, the two aspects of conscience. Motives are frequently discussed under the issue of procedures.

Abelson, R., & Friquegnon, M-L. *Ethics for Modern Life.* New York: St. Martin's Press, 1975, pp. 70–76, 154–158, 186, 258–262, 281–283, 357, 530.

American Medical News. "As science gains, moral dilemmas intensify." May 1, 1972, pp. 7–9.

Bornemeier, W.C. "Grandpa's Grandpa: A scenario for tomorrow." *The Chicago Tribune Magazine,* June 26, 1966. This scenario was reprinted in the *Journal of the American Medical Association.*

Frankena, W.K. *Ethics,* 2nd ed. Englewood Cliffs, NJ: Prentice-Hall, 1973, p. 114.

Little, D. "Duties of station versus duties of conscience: Are there two moralities?" In Jones, D., ed. *Private and Public Ethics.* New York: Edwin Mellen Press, 1979.

CHAPTER 14

EXAMINING THE IMPACT
OF MODES OF PRESENTATION

No matter how rational and objective we try to be in our case analysis and ethical reasoning, our emotional responses are an inevitable part of our decision making. There is even good reason, as Gilligan pointed out (Chapter 2), for us to question the validity and value of "truly rational and objective" decision making in ethical issues.

This chapter is an attempt to analyze and understand the emotional and sensory elements in our decision-making processes. These elements are many. For example, is it important whether a case is presented in standard clinical style or in a more personal and nontechnical mode? Does it make a difference whether you are dealing with a patient you have not met or with a patient you know personally? If a potentially emotional case is presented in a standard clinical way but reinforced with a color videotape of the health professional talking with the patient, would the visual image affect your analysis and response? Do language and style of presentation influence you?

This exercise should help you become more sensitive to the different ways in which a case is presented and the ways in which these different modes of presentation might affect your decisions.

A Case of Inappropriate Resuscitation

The question of when cardiopulmonary resuscitation is ethically appropriate is an extremely sensitive issue today. Because it is so sensitive, it often triggers very strong emotional responses whenever it is discussed. Realizing this fact, it should be obvious that the way in which this issue is presented and discussed can very easily affect one's response. A strongly worded, bluntly stated presentation will naturally trigger strong reactions. Certain phrases can even serve as "red flags," drawing a very negative or a very positive response. But this depends also on the context in which the presentation is made. An editorial format allows the presenter freedom to explore personal reactions and feelings that might be inappropriate in a research paper. What might be tolerated as a personal viewpoint in a professional newsletter might be totally unacceptable in a professional journal.

Such is the situation with the case presentation selected for analysis here. The original version, published in a professional newsletter, is bluntly worded and strongly argued (Whitacre, 1980). The language used calls forth strong reactions from the reader. A comparison is made between inappropriate resuscitation and rape. All of this was intentional on the part of the author. The tone was softened somewhat in a revised version published later in the journal *Respiratory Care* (Whitacre, 1981).

The objective of the original version, reprinted here, was not just to discuss the issue of inappropriate resuscitation but to present it in a way that would make it impossible for the reader to avoid becoming personally involved and committed to action. Whitacre's goal was to stir the reader's strongest moral condemnation of what he views as an outrageous and totally unethical medical procedure. If enough respiratory therapists and other health workers become sensitized to this issue, he hoped, it might be possible to press for recognition and for resolution of the problem by those with the power to make the change, that is, physicians and hospital administrators.

Whitacre, as a member of the health care team who is regularly called upon to resuscitate patients he believes should be left to die in peace, speaks from the frustration of powerlessness. He is frustrated by what he views as culpable neglect by those in authority, who avoid making necessary decisions. Whether he achieves this goal only you, his reader, can judge. After you read the original article, we will analyze its style and language.

OLE NINCOMPOOP SAYS: HELP STAMP OUT INAPPROPRIATE RESUSCITATION!

A month or so ago, a young lady who had had two heart surgeries and a couple of [cardiac] arrests during the past two years, which resulted in hypoxic brain damage that had left her feeble-minded and with a convulsive disorder, arrested again at home one evening because of a failing pacemaker. She was resuscitated and brought into the hospital, with no oxygen in the ambulance (!! I'm *not* making this up). There, in the medical ICU, where everyone knew her from prior admissions, she arrested AGAIN about an hour later. Since she was not "red-tagged,"* we were *obliged* to resuscitate her AGAIN, and put her on a ventilator. There, she literally rotted away for 3 or 4 weeks (they had promptly fixed her pacemaker so that her heart wouldn't be able to stop again), until, in spite of Hell (which included dialysis for renal failure for over a week), she finally managed to "die."

Now if one of the male staff had jumped into her bed and raped her, this

---

*"Red-tagged" or "No Code" are standard terms indicating that the physician and the patient, or the patient's family, have agreed that in the case of cardiac or respiratory failure no emergency or intensive care treatment will be provided.

would have been regarded as a criminal assault, and everyone would have been outraged, right? But what *we* did was far more damaging physically, far more protracted, and *not one whit less immoral*. Just the same, in the eyes of our curious social system, it was OK. Some system!

Another time recently, I was privileged to attend a Code Blue* on a patient who had arrested during cobalt therapy! That was only one of a whole series of resuscitations done routinely on terminal cancer patients at that hospital.

WHY, when such patients have literally *nothing* going for them, must we be so Hell-bent on interfering with this perfectly natural process which would relieve them of their hopeless suffering? Have our physicians taken complete leave of their senses? These are outrageous prostitutions of the art and science of resuscitation.

Resuscitation is the most literally life-saving act the therapist performs. It is the noblest, loftiest, most heroic, and *should* be the most God-like thing one mortal can do for another. But everytime I am called to one of these grossly inappropriate codes, I am sick in my soul at this UN-godly, *beastly* business. The dictum that we are *required* to resuscitate ANYbody who arrests if he is untagged, no matter what's wrong with him or how long before we find him the arrest may have occurred, really sticks in my craw. It is just reckless irresponsibility of the most irrational and immoral sort.

What's behind this tragedy? NEGLECT! Nobody talked with the patient or his family about whether he (they) wanted him resuscitated if he should arrest. Doubtless the rule always to do so in the absence of a "No Code" order was put there because of the policy that nobody but a physician should make this decision. This can of course be construed as protecting non-physicians of being accused of not resuscitating a patient who was in *their* judgment non-salvagable.

But we all know of all too many instances where the doctor has specified NOTHING either way, and where the wishes of the patient or his family have NOT been explored. This situation is, of course, inescapable when there is no time; but *usually* the subject was just plain avoided because it is too unpleasant.

I think we should complain about this to our medical directors, and try to get them to use their influence on medical staffs to face this responsibility squarely, and then definitely to "red tag" or "No Code" all patients who are either (a) not regarded as salvagable, or (b) who have expressed their desire to be allowed to die in peace. Actually, hospitals could relieve doctors of some of this unpleasantry, in case (c), by making this question a part of the Admission interview with either the patient or his family.

(Reprinted with permission from Whitacre, J. "Help stamp out inappropriate resuscitation," *The Newsletter of the Missouri Society for Respiratory Therapy*, 1980, 4.)

---

*"Code Blue" is a standard medical term for calling out the MICU, or mobile intensive care unit, with complete cardiopulmonary resuscitation.

Warming Up

As a preparation for this exercise you might want to refresh your memory on some of the decision-making skills already explored. Any of the following four steps from previous chapters can be applied to the case of inappropriate resuscitation presented by the "Ole Nincompoop."

1. Identify the ethical principles you see involved in this case (see Chapter 3).

2. Identify the specific ethical values you find applicable in this case (see Chapter 4).

3. Identify the different alternatives or ways of resolving the problem presented by the Ole Nincompoop (Chapter 7).

4. Finally, you might want to list at least one main positive and one main negative ethical consequence for each of your options as a preliminary way of sorting out the different alternatives (Chapter 9).

Phase One

By the time the Ole Nincompoop admits in the fourth paragraph of his presentation that the way resuscitations are now being handled in his hospital "really sticks in my craw," you are very aware that he is strongly emotional and obviously biased. Does that mean that his concern is not valid? Do you think the way he presents the case makes it stronger, or weaker, than if he maintained a calm, objective approach?

Can you imagine how the Ole Nincompoop would sound and look if he were presenting this case at one of your clinical sessions? Would this presentation have a different impact on you if the Ole Nincompoop were a respiratory therapy student, a clinical instructor with years of seasoned experience in the ICU, or a cardiopulmonary physician? What effect would this same presentation have on you if made by your medical director instead of by a respiratory therapist?

How does gender enter into our reactions? Would this presentation have had a different impact on you if it had been made by a female health worker? Do you think you might tend to either excuse or react negatively to this presentation if it were from "an emotional female" as opposed to the identical presentation being made by "a rational and justly angry male"?

These are all very important questions because they probe the many ways we are affected by the style, language, and visual images used in presenting a case. The mode of presentation definitely affects our ethical decisions. However subconscious the effect, it is present and should be taken into account in our decision making.

In examining the mode of presentation adopted by the Ole Nincompoop, ask yourself whether you think it was effective. Do you think it achieved the response from you that the Ole Nincompoop desired? Or, did it "turn you off" to his argument? How effective do you find his comparison of inappropriate resuscitation with rape?

Next, let's take his presentation apart. Go back over the case presentation with a red pencil or highlighter and mark all the emotionally biased words, phrases, or ideas you can find in this presentation. Include in your listing those words, phrases, or ideas that are striking for their shock value. If your instructor assigns this case for analysis, you can transfer these emotionally biased phrases to the proper place in Phase One of the exercise for this chapter in Part Two.

Phase Two

Having identified and examined the emotionally biased and shock-value phrases used by the Ole Nincompoop, you can turn his presentation completely around in two ways. You can reverse the bias and rewrite the case presentation in the same emotionally biased way to support resuscitation as long as any life remains. Or, you can rewrite the presentation by presenting Whitacre's conclusion in purely objective, unbiased terms.

For this rewrite, concentrate on the first five paragraphs of the presentation, since these contain the essence of his argument. If this case is assigned to you for analysis with the exercise form in Part Two, you will find space there for your rewritten version of the "Ole Nincompoop." If a different case is assigned, do this rewrite on a separate sheet of paper.

Phase Three

In the *Respiratory Care* version of his paper, Whitacre proposes some practical, if equally strong-worded, comments on what he believes constitutes an appropriate candidate for resuscitation. His comments are reprinted below along with a table showing a classification of patients based on the feasibility of successful resuscitation (Table 14.1).

TABLE 14.1   Classification of Patients by Feasibility of Successful Resuscitation

Good Candidates	Bad Candidates	Grey Area Candidates
1. Young persons with no known terminal illnesses 2. Patients on operating, x-ray, or cardiac catheterization lab tables or in ICUs, where arrest is instantly witnessed because patient is on monitor; and where facilities, equipment, and expertise are already available, so no time is lost	1. Patients with terminal illnesses, or who have had strokes, repeated coronaries, severe neurologic disorders, or renal failure 2. Chronic lung disease patients 3. Patients who do not want to be resuscitated 4. Any patient whose arrest was not witnessed	1. Young persons with congenital anomalies or disorders, such as cystic fibrosis; persons who are severely mentally retarded or quadriplegic 2. Middle-aged persons with several ailments, even though none is regarded as terminal
3. _____ _____ 4. _____ _____	5. _____ _____ 6. _____ _____	3. _____ _____ 4. _____ _____

SOURCE: Adapted from Whitacre, J. "Inappropriate resuscitation." *Respiratory Care*, 1981, 26(8), pp. 764–765.

INAPPROPRIATE RESUSCITATION

This can, of course, be construed as a protection for nonphysicians from the legal consequences of not resuscitating a patient they consider nonsalvageable.

However, we all know of all too many instances in which the doctor had specified nothing either way and the wishes of the patient or his family had not been explored. These situations are, of course, inescapable when there is no time; but usually the subject has been avoided because it is just too unpleasant.

I think we should complain about this to our medical directors, and try to get them to use their influence on medical staffs to face this responsibility squarely, by ordering "red tag" or "no code" designations for those patients (a) who are not regarded as salvageable, or (b) who have expressed their desire to be allowed to die in peace. Actually, hospitals could relieve doctors of some of this unpleasantry in case (b) by making this question of whether to resuscitate a part of the admission interview with the patient or his family.

To provoke discussion, Table 1 shows a proposed rough classification of patients with respect to the feasibility of successful resuscitation. I believe there should be no question whatever about whether we should resuscitate the "good" candidates: they've got lots going for them. They are the ones we should logically "pull out all the stops" for. Similarly, I believe there is no question that the "bad" ones—especially the unwitnessed ones—need a good letting alone, so that nature can help them out of a bad scene. It is seldom that the unwitnessed ones escape such cerebral anoxia that they are ever able to think again, and so it is too big a gamble for us to interfere. This leaves the "grey area" candidates, or their families if the patients are too ill or emotionally unstable, as the ones with whom it is particularly important to discuss resuscitation.

It is customary to discuss surgical procedures with patients, to acquaint them with the risks and possible sequelae involved, and to get their permission before going ahead. It does not seem fair to fail to explore the matter of resuscitation in general with patients or their families, and to fail in particular to disclose to them the possibilities of such ominous complications as the aspiration pneumonia, the pneumo- or hemothorax from broken or cracked ribs, the fat emboli and the strokes that are fairly common. If the matter comes up at all, the patient and his family are too often allowed to believe it will turn out as it does on TV, where a few good puffs, a few compressions, and a good zap with the defibrillator will have the old codger chasing nurses down the hall again in 15 or 20 minutes. How many codes have you assisted at, where the patient opened his eyes, smiled at the rescuer, and everything was hunkydory, just like in the old Heart Association CPR training films? The glamour is deceitfully played up; the gruesome, suppressed. If patients and their families had any idea what they were likely to be letting themselves in for, I'll bet darn few would opt for resuscitation, with its fruitless 10 or 20 extra hospital days, at an added cost of, say, $15,000.

We are forced to resuscitate far too many bad candidates who we can be pretty sure will never be able to think and express their personalities again. It is my contention that this is not only a disservice, it is morally criminal to inflict on an innocent person an imprisonment in a body that's alive but has a brain only partially functional—and this imprisonment, mind you, often directly against the patient's wishes had he been consulted.

All right, what can therapists do about this? Well, aside from the suggestion I've already made about urging medical directors to stop other doctors from this dereliction of responsibility, I feel there's no reason we should not talk with the patients or their families ourselves. After all, many are the times we are at the bedside with anxious relatives, who ask us, in the absence of the doctor, whether we think the patient will pull through. This is the logical time to bring the matter up. Instead of a trite answer like "who can say?" it would be smart to ask the family members whether they have discussed resuscitation with the doctor. Usually they haven't, but whether they have or not, this is the best time to advise the relatives that unless the patient has been red-tagged, he must be resuscitated, regardless of whether that is what either he or they desire. That warning alone should galvanize them into contacting the physician right away to get his counsel and to relay their wishes, so that he can write appropriate orders. While you're talking with the family members, although blowing things out of proportion regarding complications should be avoided, it is not at all inappropriate for you to give them some idea of the hideously cruel 3-ring circus they will let their loved one in for if they request that we pull out all the stops. Remind them we're perfectly willing to let him die in peace, if they just say the word.

One other thing we therapists should be doing is conducting general public education campaigns, by whatever means possible, about "living wills," whereby persons can specifically prohibit us from resuscitating them. (It's true that not many states recognize a living will yet, but the more we talk it up, the sooner more states may be pressured into passing legislation that will.) Patients who do not want to be resuscitated should advise all relatives, doctors, and hospital authorities of that fact, should wear bracelets or necklaces bearing that instruction, and should use every other possible avenue to make it generally known. Once that is done, the act of resuscitation would be more apt to be regarded as a legal assault, and after a few doctors or hospitals are sued for these inappropriate or unwanted resuscitations, I think the wishes of the individual will be more widely solicited and respected.

And that would allow us to concentrate more effort on the good candidates on whom heroics will not be so likely to backfire and produce tragic results.

(Reprinted with permission from *Respiratory Care.* Copyright 1981 by the American Association for Respiratory Therapy.)

Identify and highlight those adjectives or phrases in this excerpt that you find particularly emotional or biased. Which adjectives or phrases used here by Whitacre are effective? Which have a negative impact on you?

Delete from Table 14.1 those patients you believe should not be included in the category in which Whitacre places them. In the space below the table, add the types of patients you think should be included under any of the three categories.

Whenever you encounter a situation in which you are required to make a decision, whether or not it involves ethics, it is always helpful to examine the way in which the problem is presented to you and your reaction to this mode of presentation as it relates to your decision.

Applying This Exercise to Other Cases

Your instructor may assign the "Ole Nincompoop" case for you to analyze with the exercise form in Part Two, or a different case may be presented orally or in combination with media in class. In the latter situation, the same exercise form can be used for analysis, with a few modifications. If a film is used in presenting the case, you may be asked to identify those images that are particularly emotionally evocative, either in a positive or negative way, and to analyze their effect on your decision. Instead of describing the criteria or patient groups suitable for resuscitation, you may be asked to devise a similar list of appropriate and inappropriate candidates for some other medical procedure. In this event, the instructions given in class will be important to your proper completion of the exercise.

REFERENCES AND FURTHER READINGS

Janis, I.L., & Mann, L. *Decision Making: A Psychological Analysis of Conflict, Choice, and Commitment.* New York: Free Press, 1977, pp. 155–165, 344–367, 387–396, 424–425, 440–443.

Whitacre, J. "Ole Nincompoop says: Help stamp out inappropriate resuscitation." *Newsletter of the Missouri Society for Respiratory Therapy*, 1980, 4, pp. 11–12.

Whitacre, J. "Inappropriate resuscitation." *Respiratory Care*, 1981, 26(8), pp. 764–765. Readers responses can be found in *Respiratory Care*, 1981, 26(12), pp. 1231–1248.

CHAPTER 15
CONSENSUS DECISIONS FOR PUBLIC POLICIES

In the 1972 Broadway musical and film *1776,* Benjamin Franklin and John Adams argue the vote-trading pressure from South Carolina and Virginia that threatened to scuttle the adoption of the Declaration of Independence. The southern states refused to vote for the Declaration unless Adams agreed to withdraw the condemnation of slavery. Adams firmly believed he could never compromise his moral principle that all humans were equal and had a right to be free. While agreeing with Adams' ethical principle, Franklin was more pragmatic. He neatly analyzed the conflict of values when he remarked, in effect, that "in a democracy, decisions of importance are born of 50% compromise and 50% conviction." Franklin does not deny the principle of human equality and freedom, but in late June, 1776, he asks Adams to give priority to independence from England. After winning the first struggle, they could then press for the abolition of slavery.

Decisions made by group consensus are almost always a balance between personal compromise and group commitment. Unanimity is a luxury we seldom enjoy in group decisions. Rarely do all members of a group hold the same values, weigh them the same way, and agree unanimously on a course of action. (Hence the simplistic appeal of dictators.) Paternalistic physicians, presumed to be ultimate authorities on both medicine and morals, appeal to some patients because they absolve the patient of the responsibility for making decisions. Health care, in this context, is simple, unambiguous, and above all efficient. The physician decides; the patient accepts.

In recent years, there has been an increasing trend to make the individual patient the ultimate, autonomous arbitrator. While everyone in a health care situation has decisions to make, such decisions are subordinate to and part of the patient's decision on his or her treatment and future.

In accepting responsibility for the final decision, a patient goes through five stages implicit in all the previous chapters. First, the patient faces a challenge from his or her body by a disease or malfunction of some sort: "What are the risks if I do nothing? If the risks are too great, then I have to decide on some course of action." Having decided that action is needed, one must identify and survey the alternatives for action, such as the kinds of medication or surgery available. Then these alternatives must be weighed. In the process of weighing

173

the alternatives, the patient also makes a commitment to what appears to be the best alternative. Finally, despite the negative consequences, the patient makes a decision and commitment to act (Janis & Mann, 1977).

In institutional or social policies that depend on a consensus decision involving several people, these same five stages can be observed. Each member of the group works through the five stages. Some may move very quickly to a personal decision, whereas others will be trying to decide whether action is even necessary. Once the majority has decided some action is needed, a consensus involving some personal compromises must be reached.

One advantage of the group decision process is that it is usually more vigilant in identifying and weighing both challenges and alternatives. At least a few people in the group will question the need to change or the risks involved. Hospital ethics committees and task forces responsible for decisions on needs and resource allocations usually have established procedures for gathering and weighing information on alternatives. With members free to draw on their own fields of expertise and experience, a carefully constructed committee raises the quality of the decision making. The improved quality of group decisions has its cost in the increased time and energy required for discussion and compromise and the lost efficiency of having a "benevolent dictator." But when an issue of institutional or social policy affecting hundreds of people is in question, the experience and perspective of staff and outside physicians, allied health professionals, social workers, clergy, psychologists, and consumer advocates more than balances the loss in efficiency. A well-structured committee is more likely to identify and explore all the relevant alternatives than an individual. Ideas are exchanged and challenged, tested and weighed.

Ideal as the group process may sound, Janis and Mann are realistic in pointing out that too often "the potential advantages of group decision making are seldom realized, because conformity pressures within the group often foster a pattern of defensive avoidance among the members—a kind of 'groupthink'— rather than vigilance" (1977, p. 180). However, once a group has moved to the last two stages and made its commitment to a particular option, the new course of action is stronger than if the decision rested in the hands of a single person.

Health care professionals may or may not agree with the patient's decision on the course of treatment, depending on whether or not the decision agrees or conflicts with their own personal or professional values. Both the patient and the health professional have the right to cancel their implied social contract, as we saw in Chapter 6. In a democratic decision, on the other hand, everyone is bound by the decision. Each person has one vote. When the votes are counted and the issue decided on the basis of a simple majority, a plurality, a two-thirds majority, or some other fraction of the votes cast, the issue is settled for all.

The ethics of this democratic procedure have been debated since the days of Plato and Socrates. If the goal is the well-being of the community as a whole, and the social well-being depends on the level of individual welfare, then we have to be unanimous in our decisions. If the vote is unanimous, then everyone is convinced that he or she is not harmed by the decision and someone benefits by it. In 1776, the southern states insisted that any decision to declare independence from England had to be unanimous, knowing that at least one of the 13 colonies would veto the move. When one individual in the committee holds veto power, decisions are often impossible. Stagnation results, though a decision is still made by default: a decision not to act is nevertheless a decision. But if unanimous decisions are nearly impossible, then what of the moral dilemma between compromise and commitment? Was Adams wrong in agreeing to delay consideration of the abolition of slavery in favor of winning independence?

Kenneth Arrow, author of *Social Choice and Individual Values* (1951), and others (Hill et al., 1978) have devoted considerable attention to the inescapable problems and dilemmas of social decisions and democratic committees. When the individuals of a group each have their unique preferences, the problem is one of reconciling these varied preferences with the group decision. Arrow began by stating several plausible criteria for social decisions and examining their implications. He then demonstrated that it is impossible for a society to choose among alternatives without violating at least one of these criteria. However we may feel about Arrow's conclusions, he has addressed some of the oldest and toughest questions a free society faces. His conclusion is not an easy one to swallow, but it seems undeniable that it is impossible to arrive at a group choice in a democratic society without violating at least one of the criteria that one might expect to hold in any democracy. "Since group decisions are made in our society with less than unanimous approval, this result should alert each of us to the fact that social gains can mean losses, possibly terribly damaging ones to certain individuals" (Hill et al., 1978, p. 118).

Three Case Studies in Reproductive Technology: Variations on a Theme for Jury Decision

In this section you will find three case studies, which can be used in class for a committee or group decision exercise. When the group has decided which of the three cases it wants to debate, it can create several options or alternatives as ways of resolving the ethical issues posed by the chosen case. One or more advocates for each alternative can volunteer, be chosen by ballot, or appointed. These steps should be done before the case is presented for discussion and decision. This gives the advocates time to research and prepare their cases for presentation in class to the committee. In their presentation, the advocates for each alternative argue and defend their case. Members of the "jury" should be free to ask whatever questions they wish of the advocates.

TABLE 15.1 Comparison of First and Second Choices of Options

| Option | Percentage of Committee Members Voting | | |
	First Choice	Second Choice	Combined First and Second Choice
1	27	3	15
2	24	63	43.5
3	24	16	20
4	24	18	21

Rules for the committee decision need to be spelled out and agreed to beforehand. If more than two options are to be discussed and voted on, decide what percentage will decide the case—a simple majority, a plurality, a two-thirds vote, or other.

If several options are to be voted on, a decision should be made as to whether the committee will be allowed to express a first and second choice of options. If, for example, the vote is limited to a first choice and four options are voted on, the committee vote might turn out as follows: Option 1, 27%; option 2, 24%; option 3, 24%; option 4, 24%. If you go beyond the first choice and ask for a second preference, you might find that most of the advocates of options 3 and 4 favor option 2 as their second most ethical choice. Taking into consideration the second preference, you could have the situation shown in Table 15.1. Taking into consideration both first and second choices, the committee decision in this example clearly favors the second option instead of the first. When you have multiple options in a group decision and do not take into consideration second choices, the simple plurality vote limited to a single first choice raises a serious problem and conflict Arrow urges us to consider.

Whatever rules and criteria the committee agrees to, in the end all members must reach a consensus and make a decision. While this approach to decision making is much less structured than those outlined in previous chapters, it has its own particular value, especially when, after reaching a consensus, the committee or a couple of observers tries to analyze what occurred in the decision-making process.

CASE STUDY 1: A BILL TO REGULATE
THE USE OF SURROGATE MOTHERS

Artificial insemination was first used by Spallanzani in 1776 to produce animal offspring without benefit of sexual intercourse. Human semen was first used to artificially impregnate a woman around 1800 in England. The world's first successful human embryo transplant resulted in the birth of a daughter on July 25, 1978, to Mrs. Lesley Brown. In 1982, Mrs. Brown had a second child by embryo transplant, again using her husband's semen for "test-tube fertilization." In Australia, one woman gave birth to twins after her "test-tube fertilized" eggs were implanted in her womb to bypass blocked fallopian tubes. As of late 1983, several fertility clinics in the United States, England, Australia, Germany, and France offered embryo transplant services to married women with blocked fallopian tubes.

Meanwhile, artificial insemination with the husband's semen is increasingly being used to impregnate surrogate mothers, women who volunteer or are paid to carry a child for a couple when the wife cannot conceive or carry a pregnancy to term. At surrogate mother clinics in Philadelphia and Louisville, women prone to miscarriage can hire other women to serve as "prenatal wet nurses." These women are artificially inseminated with the husband's semen and give up the newborn infant to the couple. In some cases, single women and gay men have hired surrogate mothers in order to have a child to raise. As of January 1983, over 120 women have benefited from embryo transplants using their own ova and their husband's semen. How many couples have benefited from using surrogate mothers is anyone's guess.

A STEP TOWARD LEGAL REGULATION

On October 26, 1981, Richard Fitzpatrick, a member of the Michigan House of Representatives, introduced House Bill No. 5184, a bill to regulate surrogate parenting, with the following statement:

> The legislation I am introducing today will not introduce surrogate parenting to Michigan; it will simply regulate it.
>
> Surrogate mothering is already a reality in Michigan—and has been since at least 1976. Every month contracts are signed and inseminations are made. Every month infertile couples seek one final chance to have a child that is biologically linked to them.
>
> There are no references to surrogate parenting in the laws of the United States, Michigan, or any other state in the Union. Thus it has been assumed by some that surrogate parenting is illegal; clearly there is a need for legal guidelines and structure for the process:
>
> - Surrogate parenting without this legislation does not protect a surrogate (mother) from being misled as to the full consequences of her contract as a surrogate;
>
> - Surrogate parenting without this legislation does not protect the right of an adopting couple to be certain that the child will be theirs;
>
> - Surrogate parenting without this legislation does not guarantee that the child will have a secure and certain family structure from the moment of birth.
>
> The possibility of surrogate motherhood does not reflect any conscious public policy decision to outlaw the practice; instead it is the unintended consequence of laws regulating altogether different situations.

Surrogate mothering is growing in popularity because it meets the urgently felt needs of those who resort to it better than any other alternative they see. Subject to reasonable regulation, it deserves to take a place among the growing array of methods available to individuals for the control of their marital and reproductive lives.

I am not asking the Michigan Legislature to take a position in favor of surrogate mothering. I ask only to prevent laws created for other circumstances from eliminating this option. There is no rational reason the state should prevent a couple and a willing surrogate from participating in a legal contract. This bill, HB 5184, in addition to House Bill 4906 that I have already introduced, will simply make the law deal with the reality that is already existing across the state.

ISSUE

Should a law be passed regulating surrogate parenting, and if so, what kind of a law? What should its details and restrictions be?

CASE STUDY 2: SELECTIVE ABORTION

This ethical situation (Kerenyi & Chitkara, 1981) arose in 1981 when a New England woman in her 30s became pregnant with twins. Because of the woman's age, amniocentesis was recommended in the seventeenth week of pregnancy. Ultrasound scanning allowed safe sampling of the amniotic fluid from each fetus. It was discovered that one fetus suffered from Down's syndrome whereas the other twin was normal.

Physicians guided a needle into the heart of the fetus with Down's syndrome and withdrew a quarter of its blood. The risk to the normal fetus was considered minimal because of the careful use of ultrasound scanning. The Down's fetus, who died as a result of the removal of blood, was carried to term. Shortly after the delivery of the normal twin, the mother delivered the fragile, paper-thin, nonliving fragments of the defective twin, a fetus papyraceus.

While the recurrence of such situations is likely to be very rare, the question of selective abortion of one fetus in a multiple pregnancy is one that will continue to arise.

ISSUE

Is the selective abortion of one fetus in a multiple pregnancy ethical, and if so, under what circumstances would it be ethical (e.g., if the fetus were of an undesired gender or mentally or genetically handicapped)?

CASE STUDY 3: MATERNAL REFUSAL
OF TREATMENT THREATENS FETAL LIFE

A young woman who was a Jehovah's Witness, had been informed by her physician that the 3-month-old fetus she was carrying suffered from a severe anemia that could result in the fetus being stillborn or mentally retarded. After discussing the case with the physician and consulting with her religious leaders, the woman decided that God had wanted her to bear the child with this problem. Her conviction that prenatal transfusion and the surgery necessary to increase the chances of giving birth to a normal, healthy child would be immoral and contrary to her religious faith was carefully reasoned and firm. The physician felt she had a moral obligation to the fetus she was carrying. When he could not convince her, he took the case to court seeking an order that would force the woman to allow the prenatal transfusion and surgery. When the woman learned that the court had ordered the transfusion despite her religious protest, she fled the state.

ISSUE

The courts have traditionally ordered blood transfusions and surgery to save the lives of minors when parents refuse to approve such procedures on the grounds that they violate religious beliefs. Should the court extend this protection to the fetus early in pregnancy, and if so, under what circumstances?

Applying the Consensus Approach
to Making Decisions on Public Policy

The three brief case studies above revolve around the growing issues of fetal engineering and reproductive technology. While the area of human reproduction has traditionally been viewed as a sacred, inviolate, private domain of the couple and of the pregnant woman, medical technology poses new, disturbing questions that bring these issues into the domain of public policy and social concern. The tensions between the private and social domains are now unavoidable, as are the emotionally charged debates they trigger.

The exercise in Part Two is to be used in conjunction with a committee decision on one of the three cases outlined above. The instructor may, however, assign a different case more applicable to local interests or to a current event. The exercise will help you structure the committee's deliberations and analyze the proceedings.

REFERENCES AND FURTHER READINGS

Arrow, K.J. *Social Choice and Individual Values.* New York: John Wiley & Sons, 1951.

Hill, P., et al. *Making Decisions: A Multidisciplinary Introduction.* Reading, MA: Addison-Wesley, 1979, pp. 115–119.

Janis, I., & Mann, L. *Decision Making: A Psychological Analysis of Conflict, Choice, and Commitment.* New York: Free Press, 1977, pp. 109–120, 129–133, 174–180, 295–401.

Jonsen, A.R., & Butler, L.H. "Public ethics and policy making." *Hastings Center Report,* 1975, *5*(4), pp. 19–31.

Kerenyi, T.D., & Chitkara, U. "Selective abortion of a Downs' syndrome twin." *New England Journal of Medicine,* 1981, *304*(25), pp. 1525–1527.

Neville, R. "On the National Commission: A Puritan critique of consensus ethics." *Hastings Center Report,* 1979, *9*(2), pp. 22–27.

Purtilo, R.B., & Cassel, C.K. *Ethical Dimensions in the Health Professions.* Philadelphia: W.B. Saunders, 1981, pp. 161–180.

Robertson, J.A. "Ten ways to improve IRBs." *Hastings Center Report,* 1979, *9*(1), pp. 29–33.

Veatch, R.M. "Institutional review boards: The National Commission recommendations on IRBs." *Hastings Center Report,* 1979, *9*(1), pp. 22–28.

NOTES

CHAPTER 16

THE ULTIMATE QUESTION: WHO IS A PERSON, AND WHY?

As a final exercise in this worktext, we return to the two world views discussed in Chapter 1. We began by contrasting two ends of the spectrum in cosmologies, with the fixed philosophy of nature on one end leading to a duty-oriented view of ethics, and the process view of the world on the other end inclining toward a consequence-oriented approach to ethics. Some ethicists have suggested that recent developments in fetology, coma rehabilitation, and thanatology are pressing both the duty-oriented and the consequence-oriented ethicists to refine and sharpen their arguments in a way that will eventually lead to a convergence of the more moderate advocates on both ends of the continuum. "We find that these approaches, which at times seemed so divergent and antipathetic, [increasingly] appear to borrow from each other and end up saying the same thing" (Barton, 1965).

The focus in all biomedical ethics is the person, the being who claims the personal rights and bears the personal responsibilities discussed in our previous chapters. The ultimate question in biomedical ethics, then, can be phrased in several ways. How do we ascertain who qualifies as a person? What criteria or characteristics tell us this status has been achieved? When does someone cease to be a person? On what basis do we decide that this status has been lost? These intertwined questions have provoked heated debate throughout human history. In the past, our operational definitions of personhood have, at one time or another, excluded women, blacks, American Indians, the Incas and Mayans, and others.

Today, in modern medicine, politics, and religion questions of the nature of personhood and the debate they provoke are even more challenging. Although they may prove to be unanswerable questions, we still must face them. At least we can try to devise an operational definition of the human person that is more realistic and in tune with our current knowledge than those that have been used until now in our biomedical ethical decisions. Such a new and more realistic operational definition is desperately needed.

The abortion debate is the most obvious situation in which we need a new definition of the human person. Those who adhere to a fixed philosophy of nature and duty-oriented ethics often hold that a person with full, absolute human rights exists from the moment of fertilization, or from the time of conception or uterine implantation, about 4 or 5 days after fertilization. Some, like Ramsey, claim that the fetus is a person once the embryonic disk is no longer capable of dividing into identical twins, somewhere in the second week after fertilization. A few are inclined to follow the medieval principle of "quickening," when the woman begins to feel definite movements of the fetus in her womb, usually in the fourth month of pregnancy. In the past, some cultures placed the time of attaining personhood at birth, or even 8 days after birth when, if the infant survived, it was given a name and, if a boy, was circumcised. The question is whether any absolutist, all-or-nothing view of personhood can be reconciled with current knowledge of embryology, neurophysiology, and the whole of modern science, which is based on a process or developmental view of nature that includes human nature (Francoeur, 1977).

The ultimate question also arises when reproduction specialists fertilize four or five eggs taken from a woman with blocked fallopian tubes but implant only one of the resultant embryonic masses in her womb. If the remaining embryonic masses are discarded or frozen for later use in other infertile women, what is their status as persons?

McNulty (1981) and Andrews (1981) reported an unusual attempt by Chinese scientists to fertilize a chimpanzee egg with human sperm to produce a "near-human ape." This creature, it was suggested, could work at routine jobs, herd sheep and cows, and drive carts. It could be used as a living bank of organs for transplants. It might be useful in exploring space or the ocean floors and in mines. What would be the personhood status of such a creature?

The increasing use of prenatal monitoring, our early ventures into human genetic engineering, and our growing ability to operate on the fetus in the womb add to the necessity of our reexamining the traditional definitions of personhood.

Finally there is the challenge posed by the work of Robert L. White, at Case Western Reserve Medical School, and by others in the "experimental transference of consciousness" with monkeys and the possibility of creating a "human equivalent." In the opening sentence of his 1978 report to the Seventh International Conference on the Unity of Science in Boston, White pointed out that "in recent years we have been able to construct a series of brain models which have permitted us to literally transfer the entire brain of the experimental animal [a monkey] intact and still capable of high performance at all levels." In closing his report, White reminds us that "science has reached the threshold where *human consciousness can be transferred* provided the organ which supervenes this characteristic is maintained. Whether research directed toward human cephalic transplantation should be undertaken requires extensive review by such fields as philosophy, theology, sociology, and medicine" (White, 1978).

In the 1980s research such as this will make it impossible for us to ignore the necessity of a new operational definition of personhood as a basis for our discussions of dilemmas in biomedical ethics. Yet the difficulties of reaching a consensus on a new operational definition cannot be overstated at a time when the rift between fundamentalist and process thinking is becoming more evident and explosive. Even if we managed to achieve agreement on such a new operational definition, it will take us decades to resolve the philosophical, theological, and legal implications it would pose. Real as they are, these difficulties should not deter us. For this reason the final chapter in this worktext is a tentative excursion into the decision-making process related to developing a contemporary and realistic operational definition of personhood.

Developing a Process-Oriented Operational Definition of Personhood

Ten years ago, Joseph Fletcher recognized our need for a new developmental operational definition of the human person. Fletcher's experience gave him a broad perspective from which to work. As a young minister during the Great Depression of the 1930s, he had worked in the slums of London. In 1936, he was appointed graduate dean of a seminary in Cincinnati. In 1944, he became professor of theology and Christian ethics at the Episcopal Theological School in Cambridge, Massachusetts. More recently, he has been a visiting professor of medical ethics at the University of Virginia School of Medicine.

Morals and Medicine, Fletcher's 1954 exploration of contraception, artificial insemination, sterilization, euthanasia, and the patient's right to be informed, is still an important reference. In 1966, Fletcher added a whole new dimension to our ethical thinking with his provocative description and delineation of situation ethics.

Always deeply involved in issues of medical and sexual ethics, Fletcher tackled the problem of redefining human personhood in 1972 with a challenging watershed paper presented at the National Conference on the Teaching of Medical Ethics. To provide a solid basis for our exercise in redefining the nature of personhood, an adapted version of Fletcher's 1972 paper is reproduced here. Notice, as you read it, his description of the need for a new definition and the careful way he proposes his tentative profile of personhood. Later, in the exercise for this chapter, you are asked to react in a critical way to his specific suggestions of new criteria for personhood. You will also be asked to rank or weight his criteria for personhood status.

FLETCHER'S "INDICATORS OF HUMANHOOD"

Mark Twain complained that people are always talking about the weather but they never do anything about it. The same is true of the humanhood agenda. In biomedical ethics, writers constantly say that we need to explicate humanness, or humaneness—what it means to be a truly human being—but they never follow their admission of the need with an actual inventory or profile, no matter how tentatively offered.

Synthetic concepts such as *human* and *man* and *person* require operational terms, spelling out the which and what and when. Only in that way can we get down to cases—to normative decisions. There are always some people who prefer to be visceral and affective in their moral choices, with no desire to have any rationale for what they do. But *ethics* is precisely the business of rational, critical reflection (encephalic and not merely visceral) about the problems of the moral agent—in biology and medicine as much as in law, government, education or anything else.

To that end, then, for the purposes of biomedical ethics, I am suggesting a "profile of personhood" in concrete and discrete terms. As only one person's reflection on personhood, it will no doubt invite adding and subtracting by others, but this is the road to be followed if we mean business. As a dog is said to "worry" a bone, let me worry out loud and on paper, hoping for some agreement and, at the least, consideration. I have suggested fifteen positive and five negative propositions. Since there is space only to itemize and not to explain in detail, let me set them out, in no rank order at all, and as hardly more than a list of criteria or indicators.

Positive Human Criteria

Minimal Intelligence: Any individual of the species *Homo sapiens* who falls below the I.Q. 40-mark in a standard Stanford-Binet test, amplified if you like by other tests, is questionably a person; below the 20-mark, not a person. The *ratio* [reasoning], in another turn of speech, is what makes a person of the *vita* [living being]. Mere biological life, before minimal intelligence is achieved or after it is lost irretrievably, is without personal status. This has bearing, obviously, on decision making in gynecology, obstetrics, and pediatrics, as well as in general surgery and medicine.

Self-awareness: Self-consciousness, as we know, is the quality we watch developing in a baby; we watch it with fascination and glee. Its essential role in personality development is a basic datum of psychology. Its existence or function in animals at or below the primate level (of monkeys, chimpanzees, and apes) is debatable; it is clearly absent in the lower vertebrates, as well as in the nonvertebrates. In psychotherapy, non-self-awareness is pathological; in medicine, unconsciousness when it is incorrigible at once poses quality-of-life judgments—for example, in neurosurgical cases of irreversible damage to the brain cortex.

Self-control: If an individual is not only not controllable by others (unless by force) but not controllable by the individual himself or herself, a low level of life is reached about on a par with a paramecium. If the condition cannot be rectified medically, so that means-to-an-end behavior is out of the question, the individual is not a person—not ethically, and certainly not in the eyes of the law—just as a fetus is not legally a person.

A Sense of Time: Time consciousness. A sense, that is, of the passage of time. A colleague of mine at the University of Virginia, Dr. Thomas Hunter, remarked recently, ''Life is the allocation of time.'' We can disagree legitimately about how relatively important this indicator is, but it is hard to understand why anybody would minimize it or eliminate it as a trait of humanness.

A Sense of Futurity: How ''truly human'' is any individual who cannot realize there is a time yet to come as well as a present? Subhuman animals do not look forward in time; they live only on what we call visceral strivings, appetites. Philosophical anthropologies commonly emphasize *purposiveness* as a key to humanness. Chesterton once remarked that we would never ask a puppy what manner of dog it wanted to be when it grows up. The assertion here is that persons are typically teleological [oriented towards goals], although certainly not all are eschatological [looking to a life after death].

A Sense of the Past: Memory. Unlike other animals, persons as a species have reached a unique level of neurologic development, particularly the cerebrum and especially its neo-cortex. They are linked to the past by conscious recall— not only, as with subhumans, by conditioning and the reactivation of emotions (reactivated, that is, externally rather than autonomously). It is this trait, in particular, that makes persons, alone among all species, a cultural instead of an instinctive creature. An existentialist focus on ''nowness'' truncates the nature of people.

The Capability to Relate to Others: Inter-personal relationships, of the sexual-romantic and friendship kind, are of the greatest importance for the fullness of what we idealize as being truly personal. (Medical piety in the past has always held its professional ethics to be only a one-to-one, physician-patient obliga-tion.) However, there are also the more diffuse and comprehensive social re-lations of our vocational, economic, and political life. Aristotle's characterization of humans as social animals, *zoon politicon*, must surely figure prominently in the inventory. It is true that even insects live in social systems, but the cohesion of all subhuman societies is based on instinct. Human society is based on cul-ture—that is, on a conscious knowledge of the system and on the exercise in some real measure of either consent or opposition.

Concern for Others: Some people may be skeptical about our capacity to care about others (what in Christian ethics is often distinguished from romance and friendship as "fraternal love" or "neighborly concern"). The extent to which this capacity is actually in play is debatable. But whether concern for others is interested in or inspired by enlightened self-interest it seems plain that a con-scious extra-ego orientation is a trait of the species; the absence of this ambience is a clinical indication of psychopathology.

Communication: Utter alienation or disconnection from others, if it is irrepar-able, is de-humanization. This is not so much a matter of not being disposed to receive and send "messages" as it is of the inability to do so. This criterion comes into question in patients who cannot hear, speak, feel or see others; it may come about as a result of mental or physical trauma, infection, genetic or congenital (birth) disorder, or from psychological causes. Completely and finally *isolated* individuals are subpersonal. The problem is perhaps most familiar in terminal illnesses and the clinical decision-making required.

Control of Existence: It is of the nature of people that they are not helplessly subject to the blind workings of physical or physiological nature. They have only finite knowledge, freedom, and initiative, but what they possess is real and effective. Invincible ignorance and total helplessness are the antithesis of humanness, and to the degree that a person lacks control he or she is not responsible, and to be irresponsible is to be subpersonal. This applies directly, for example, in psychiatric medicine, especially to severe cases of toxic and degenerative psychosis.

Curiosity: To be without affect, sunk in anomie, is to be not a person. Indif-ference is inhuman. A person is a learner and a knower as well as a tool maker and user. This raises a question, therefore, about demands to stop some kinds of biomedical inquiry. For example, an A.M.A. committee recently called a halt to *in vitro* reproduction and embryo transplants on the grounds that they are dangerous. But dangerous ignorance is more dangerous than dangerous knowledge. It is dehumanizing to impose a moritorium on research. No doubt this issue arises, or will arise, in many other phases of medical education and practice.

Change and Changeability: To the extent that an individual is unchangeable or opposed to change he or she denies the creativity of personal beings. It means not only the fact of biological and physiological change, which is a condition of life, but the capacity and disposition for changing one's mind and conduct as well. Biologically, human beings are developmental; birth, life, health, and death are processes, not events, and are to be understood epigenetically, not episodically. All human existence is on a continuum, a matter of becoming. The question arises prominently in abortion ethics.

Balance of Rationality and Feeling: To be "truly human," to be a whole *person,* one can be neither Apollonian [purely intellectual] nor Dionysian [purely emotional]. As human beings we are not "coldly" rational or cerebral, nor are we merely creatures of feelings and intuition. It is a matter of being both, in different combinations from one individual to another. To be one rather than the other is to distort the *humanum.*

Idiosyncrasy: The human being is idiomorphous, a distinctive individual. As Helmut Schoeck has shown, even the function of envy in human behavior is entirely consistent with idiosyncrasy. To be a person is to have an identity, to be recognizable and callable by name. It is this criterion which lies behind the fear that to replicate individuals by so-called "cloning" would be to make "carbon copies" of the parent source and thus dehumanize the clone by denying its individuality. One or two writers have even spoken of a "right" to a "unique genotype," and while such talk is ethically and scientifically questionable it nonetheless reflects a legitimate notion of something essential to an authentic person.

Neo-cortical Function: In a way, this is *the cardinal indicator, the one on which all the others hinge.* Before the cerebration begins or with its end, in the absence of the synthesizing function of the cerebral cortex, the *person* is non-existent. Such individuals are objects, not subjects, no matter how many spontaneous or artificially supported functions persist in the heart, lungs, neurological and vascular systems. Such non-cerebral processes are not personal. Like the Harvard Medical School's *ad hoc* committee report on "brain death," the recent Kansas statute on defining death requires the absence of *brain* function. So do the guidelines recently adopted by the Italian Council of Ministers. But what is definitive in determining death is the loss of cerebration, not just of any or all brain function. Personal reality depends on cerebration and to be dead "humanly" speaking is to be ex-cerebral, no matter how long the *body* remains alive.

Negative Human Criteria

Five negative points can be put even more briefly than the 15 positive ones, although I am inclined to believe that they merit just as much critical scrutiny and elaboration.

Humans Are Not Non- or Anti-artificial: As Gaylin says, humans are characterized by technique, and for a human being to oppose technology is "self-hatred." We are often confused on this score, attitudinally. A "test tube baby," for example, although conceived and gestated *ex corpo*, would nonetheless be humanly reproduced and of human value. A baby made artificially, by deliberate and careful contrivance, would be *more human* than one resulting from sexual roulette—the reproductive mode of the subhuman species.

Humans Are Not Essentially Parental: People can be fully personal without reproducing, as the religious vows of nuns, monks and celibate priests of the past have asserted, as the law implied by refusing to annul marriages because of sterility, and as we see in the ethos-reversal of contemporary family and population control—and more militantly, in the non-parental rhetoric of feminists and a growing rejection of the "baby trap."

Humans Are Not Essentially Sexual: Sexuality, a broader and deeper phenomenon than sex, is of the fullness but not of the essence of personhood. It is not even necessary for species survival. I will not try to indicate the psychological entailments of this negative proposition, but it is biologically apparent when we look at such non-sexual reproduction as cloning from somatic cells, and parthenogenic reproduction [virginal conception] by both androgenesis and gynogenesis [sperm developing without union with an egg, or an egg developing without being fertilized by a sperm]. What light does this biology throw on the nature of personhood; what does a personalistic view of the human say about the ethics of such biology?

A Human Is Not a Bundle of Rights: The notion of a human *nature* has served as a conceptual bucket, to contain "human rights" and certain other *given* things, like "original sin" and "the sense of oughtness" and "conscience." The idea behind this is that such things are objective, pre-existent phenomena, not contingent on biological or social relativities. People sometimes speak of rights to live, to die, to be healthy, to reproduce, and so on, as if they were absolute, eternal, intrinsic. But as the law makes plain, all rights are imperfect and may be set aside if human *need* requires it. We shall have to think through the relation of rights and needs, as it bears on clinical medicine's decision-making problems, as well as society's problems of health care delivery. One example: What is the "humane" policy if we should reach the point (and I think we will) of deciding for or against compulsory birth control? Or, how are we to relate rights and needs if, to take only one example, an ethnic group protests mass screening for sickle cell anemia? Or if after genetic counseling a couple elects to proceed with a predictably degenerative pregnancy?

A Person Is Not a Worshiper: Faith in supernatural realities and attempts to be in direct association with them are choices some human beings make and others do not. Mystique is not essential to being truly a person. Like sexuality, it may be of the fullness of humanness but it is not necessarily of the essence. This negative proposition is required by our basic guideline, the premise that a viable biomedical ethics is humanistic, whatever reasons we may have for putting human well being at the center of concern.

More Thinking

How are we to test such criteria as these? And how are we to compare and combine the results of our criticism? *How are we to rank, order, or give priority to the items in our personhood profile?* Which are only optimal and which are essential? What are the applications of these or other indicators to the normative decisions of biologists and physicians? In my own list which factors can be eliminated, in whole or in part, without lowering individuals and patients below the personal line? I trust that by this time it is plain that I do not claim to have produced the pure gospel of humanness. I remain open to correction.

The "nature of personhood" question is of such depth and sensitivity that it is bound to raise controversy. Our task is not only to welcome the controversy but also to try to reduce it through analysis and synthesis. Heraclitus said that: "Opposition brings concord. Out of discord comes the fairest harmony. It is by disease that health is pleasant; by evil that good is pleasant; by hunger, satiety; by weariness, rest."

As a final note, I suspect that we are more apt to find good answers inductively and empirically, from medical science and the clinicians, than by the necessarily syllogistic reasoning of the humanities, which proceeds deductively from abstract premises. Syllogisms always contain their conclusions in their major or first premises. Divorced from the laboratory and the hospital, talk about what it means to be human could easily become inhumane.

(Adapted from Fletcher, J. "Indicators of humanhood: A tentative profile of man." *Hastings Center Report*, 1972, 2(5), pp. 1–4. Used with permission of the Hastings Center Report.)

Some Critical Reactions to Fletcher's Tentative Profile of Personhood

Before attempting your own analysis of Fletcher's tentative profile, it may be helpful to review some of the responses his proposal provoked from professional philosophers and ethicists.

Two years after Fletcher's paper was published, he summarized these responses (Fletcher, 1974). After repeating his contention that the most acute question in medical ethics today is our understanding of what is a *person*, Fletcher repeated his suggestion that in his 15 positive and five negative criteria, neocortical function "is the cardinal or hominizing trait upon which all the other human traits hinge." The responses suggested three other traits as the cardinal trait or singular *esse* of humaneness. In addition to neocortical function, self-consciousness, relational ability, and happiness were suggested by critics, the last being included, according to Fletcher, "more in a light than a heavy vein." The other characteristics can be described as optimal indicators, part of the fullness of personhood but not central or essential. Note that not one of the four suggested cardinal indicators or the remaining optimal traits excludes the others. They are all, more or less, part of the profile of personhood.

Nevertheless, the decisive question remains: Which of the four cardinal indicators, if any, is required in order to have the other three, and the remaining optimal indicators as well?

In commenting on Fletcher's profile, Michael Tooley, an ethicist at Stanford University, opts for self-awareness, or subjectivity, as his essential cardinal criterion. Since the human mind is not a static substance or event but a dynamic reality acquired in a developmental process, a growing fetus is a person once its neurologic "switchboard" is connected in a way that allows consciousness of self to emerge.

Richard McCormick, of Georgetown University, takes a different tack, arguing that "the meaning, substance, and consummation of life is found in human relationships." Human life, then, "is a value to be preserved only insofar as it contains some potentiality for human relationships." With this criterion, anencephalics certainly are not persons, although they are human. Individuals with an IQ below 40, in the "idiot" range, would probably lack personhood. "If that potential [for interpersonal relationships] is simply nonexistent or would be utterly submerged and undeveloped in the mere struggle to survive, that life has achieved its potential" and need not be prolonged, according to McCormick.

A pediatrician at the Texas Medical Center in Houston took strong exception to McCormick's position. "I know a little four-year-old boy," she told Fletcher, "certainly 20 minus or an idiot on any measurement scale and untrainable, but just the same he is a human being and nobody is going to tell me different. He is happy and that makes him human, as human as you or I."

Neocortical activity, the ability to relate, self-awareness, happiness—which one of these contains the essence of personhood? Tristram Engelhardt, of the Texas Medical Branch (Galveston), rejects the claim that any single criterion is sufficient. Instead, he creates an operational definition of personhood that includes three dimensions: cerebral function, self-consciousness, and a relational capacity.

In summarizing these comments, Fletcher reminds us that "neocortical death means that both self-consciousness and other-orientedness are gone." Amnesia victims, on the other hand, may have lost their self-awareness but they retain their neocortical activity. Autistic and schizophrenic persons may not be able to relate with others, but their cerebral activity and self-awareness are intact, however confused. Medically, we can ascertain the presence or absence of neocortical activity in an individual. We can also ascertain when neural integration has been impaired beyond recovery in cerebral death. The ability to relate interpersonally and the capacity or potential for self-awareness are much more difficult, or perhaps impossible, to determine. But as Fletcher concludes, the "discussion goes on."

Applying These Concepts to Your Operational Definition of Personhood

The exercise for this chapter in Part Two has been designed to make you a part of the on-going discussion of an operational definition of personhood. Recalling our discussion of two world views and two ethical systems in Chapter 1, you are asked to take both sides of the issue. First, you can develop your own defense of the human person in terms of an absolutist or fixed philosophy of nature. You can then elaborate on and defend one of the process views offered by Fletcher and his commentators.

As a final step, after reexamining carefully the 20 positive and negative criteria proposed by Fletcher, you can use the weighting techniques from Chapters 4 and 7 to assign priorities to the different indicators and perhaps even arrive at a single cardinal criterion of personhood.

This same process can be utilized in a class discussion. The class can be divided into two camps, one defending the process view of personhood and the other arguing for the absolutist view. Individual criteria in Fletcher's tentative profile can also be debated in the same way by students in the class.

REFERENCES AND FURTHER READINGS

Andrews, L. "Embryo technology." *Parents' Magazine,* 1981, *56*(5), pp. 63–71.

Barton, R.T. "Ethical systems and theory." *Journal of the American Medical Association.* 1965, *193*(2), pp. 133–138.

Ebgelhardt, H.T. "Medicine and the concept of person." In Beauchamp, T.L., & Walters, L., eds. *Contemporary Issues in Bioethics,* 2nd ed. Belmont, CA: Wadsworth, 1982, pp. 93–100.

Feinberg, J. "The problem of personhood." In Beauchamp, T.L., & Walters, L., eds. *Contemporary Issues in Bioethics,* 2nd ed. Belmont, CA: Wadsworth, 1982, pp. 108–116.

Fletcher, J. "Indicators of humanhood: A tentative profile of man." *Hastings Center Report,* 1972, 2(5), pp. 1–4. Some minor editing has been done in the version given in Chapter 16, with the author's permission, for the sake of conciseness and clarity.

Fletcher, J., et al. "Responses to a tentative profile of personhood." *Hastings Center Report,* 1973, 4(6), pp. 4–7.

Francoeur, R.T. *Utopian Motherhood: New Trends in Human Reproduction,* 3rd ed. Cranbury, NJ: A.S. Barnes Perpetua, 1977, pp. 68–82.

McNulty, T. "Chinese attempt a human-chimpanzee hybrid." *Chicago Tribune,* February 12, 1981.

Puccetti, R. "The life of a person." In Beauchamp, T.L., & Walters, L., eds. *Contemporary Issues in Bioethics,* 2nd ed. Belmont, CA: Wadsworth, 1982, pp. 101–107.

White, R.L. "Experimental transference of consciousness: The human equivalent." In *The Reevaluation of Existing Values and the Search for Absolute Values: Proceedings of the Seventh International Conference on the Unity of the Sciences,* Vol. 2. New York: International Cultural Foundation Press, 1978, pp. 705–710.

NOTES

CONCLUSION: A SYNTHESIS
OF DECISION-MAKING METHODS

CONCLUSION: A SYNTHESIS OF DECISION-MAKING METHODS

In 16 brief chapters we dissected two main themes, the levels of ethical thinking and the techniques for making decisions. We can now bring these two themes together in a brief summary. This synthesis and conclusion will have much more meaning now that you have worked your way through the chapters and exercises than it did when first sketched out in the introduction. A quick look back to the figure in the introduction, however, will refresh your visual image of where you have been.

In the first theme, we explored the four levels of ethical thinking: ethical systems, principles, rules, and decisions. On the systems level, we examined the impact of three different general continua on our ethical thinking and decisions. The two basic cosmologies or world views, the fixed philosophy of nature and the process view, the spectrum of duty-oriented versus consequence-oriented ethical systems, and the gender-based male concern with rights and female concern with relationships turned up repeatedly in our later decision-making exercises. The six basic ethical principles—personal autonomy, confidentiality, beneficence, nonmaleficence, veracity, and justice—also came to the surface time and again in our ethical rules and decisions.

The various steps and techniques of making ethical decisions, were, of course, our main theme. Global and local problems of triage, the social contract between the health worker and the patient, and identifying and sorting alternatives served as a prelude to your experience working through eight different decision-making techniques. Each of these techniques, as you now know, has its own strengths and limitations. A decision tree will work with most cases, and the consensus technique for public policies will have wide application. The quantitative analysis involved in the decision matrix and the projection of motives are techniques you may rarely use in a conscious format. The value of this manual and of your working through these various exercises and techniques is that it helps you, perhaps for the first time, become aware of the elements and factors involved in making good ethical decisions. How often you consciously use this or that technique in your personal or professional life is not important. Most of the time when you face a decision, you will not sit down with any particular exercise form you used here, although there may be times when such discipline will be useful. Most of the time, however, you will find yourself semiconsciously combining a variety of skills and sensitivities gained in your work with these exercises.

Like any beginner who takes classes in how to paint, type, or play a musical instrument, you have spent time learning basic techniques. These first learning experiences are always painful and tedious. Later, with the new skills absorbed as part of your thinking processes, you can use them to advantage, at times almost instinctively. Just as the advanced typist or skilled musician automatically uses the techniques and skills so painfully labored over in earlier days, you will find yourself applying the ethical sensitivities and decision skills gained in these 16 chapters and exercises to your everyday professional work. Gaining these abilities will enable you to express a greater sensitivity to the dignity and needs of those people you encounter in health care situations. Health care delivery thus becomes more holistic, humane, and transcendent of the limits of human egotism.

If the basic ethical principle of "doing unto others as you would have them do unto you" has any meaning in the delivery of health care, then health care workers have a life-long challenge to become ever more sensitive to and concerned about the dignity of every person who depends on them in times of emergency and need. The goal of biomedical ethics is to help us strive with greater effectiveness toward humane and holistic health care.

PART TWO
EXERCISES AND FORMS FOR APPLYING DECISION-MAKING STEPS AND TECHNIQUES

1 DUTY-ORIENTED AND CONSEQUENCE-ORIENTED THINKING

CHAPTER 1 EXERCISE
DUTY-ORIENTED AND CONSEQUENCE-ORIENTED THINKING

CASE TITLE

NAME

CLASS

Phase One

Where do you see yourself in the spectrum of ethical systems? Are you inclined toward duty or toward consequences as a basis for deciding what is right or wrong about an action? Why?

_____

_____

_____

_____

_____

_____

_____

_____

_____

_____

Which world view is more convincing to you, a world that is essentially finished and unchanging, or a world in which the very essence of things is changing and everything is in process? Why?

_____

_____

_____

_____

_____

_____

Using a case of your own choice or one assigned to you in class, identify its basic ethical problem or dilemma. To solve this problem, decide on a course of action. Something should be done or should not be done because it is the morally right or wrong action. State the ethical problem and one of the several solutions possible in the space provided. The main ethical issue in this case is

_____

_____

_____

A solution (action) that might be or was used in this case is _____

_____

_____

Phase Two

Refresh you understanding of duty-oriented thinking presented on pages 5–15 and in Figure 1.2. Create an argument for or against the proposed or actual solution you wrote above. Remember, your argument must be based on some general principle that is either revealed or deducible by reason from nature.

_____

_____

Review the explanation of consequence-oriented thinking presented on page 8 and in Figure 1.3. Then create an argument in favor of the proposed or actual solution in the case above. Remember, your argument must be based on some criteria of consequences, utility, or happiness for the majority and least harm to the fewest.

_____

_____

_____

_____

_____

_____

_____

_____

_____

_____

_____

_____

_____

_____

_____

_____

_____

_____

_____

_____

_____

_____

Again, following consequence-oriented ethical thinking, create a second argument, this time against the proposed or actual solution in this case. Your argument must be based on stronger negative consequences and harm to the majority.

_____

_____

_____

_____

_____

_____

_____

_____

_____

_____

_____

_____

_____

_____

_____

Phase Three (Optional)

Discuss with a member of the clergy, in your own religious tradition or in another tradition, the two world views and the two general ethical systems to find out where he or she fits into these two spectrums.

Outline your thoughts in rough form here before composing your final answers for this exercise.

2 GENDER-RELATED MORAL THINKING

CHAPTER 2 EXERCISE
GENDER-RELATED
MORAL THINKING

_____   _____
CASE TITLE   NAME

                                    _____
                                    CLASS

Be sure you select or are assigned a case that has as a primary factor a strong human relationship. This is necessary if you are to follow the two paths of justice/rights and caring relations. On this page and the next make some statements, opinions, and suggestions based on justice, fairness, equality, and the rights of the people involved in the case for resolving the ethical dilemma. The far right column in Table 2.1 and the comments of Jake cited in the chapter may be helpful to you in suggesting ideas and wording for these statements.

_____

_____

_____

_____

_____

_____

_____

_____

_____

_____

_____

_____

_____

_____

_____

_____

_____

_____

_____

_____

_____

_____

_____

_____

_____

_____

_____

_____

_____

_____

_____

_____

_____

_____

_____

_____

Now make some statements, opinions, and suggestions based on the responsibility of caring and the effect on the relationship in your case for solving the ethical dilemma.

_____

_____

3 IDENTIFYING ETHICAL PRINCIPLES

CHAPTER 3 EXERCISE
IDENTIFYING ETHICAL PRINCIPLES

PROFESSIONAL CODE ANALYZED

NAME

CLASS

Select one of the following professional codes of ethics for analysis or analyze the code assigned by your instructor. In the first six boxes check which of the ethical principles listed below are inherent in or supported by that statement.

1. Autonomy

2. Veracity

3. Nonmaleficence

4. Beneficence

5. Confidentiality

6. Justice

Then, rank each statement for importance in the ethical delivery of health care using a scale of 5 for very important and 1 for minimal importance.

DECLARATION OF GENEVA

Medical vow adopted by the General Assembly of The World Medical Association at Geneva, Switzerland, September 1948, and amended by the 22nd World Medical Assembly, Sydney, Australia, August 1968.

	Autonomy	Veracity	Nonmaleficence	Beneficence	Confidentiality	Justice	Rank

At the Time of Being Admitted as a Member of the Medical Profession:

I solemnly pledge myself to consecrate my life to the service of humanity.

I will give to my teachers the respect and gratitude which is their due;

I will practice my profession with conscience and dignity;

The health of my patient will be my first consideration;

I will respect the secrets which are confided in me; even after the patient has died.

I will maintain by all the means in my power, the honor and the noble traditions of the medical profession;

My colleagues will be my brothers;

I will not permit considerations of religion, nationality, race, party politics or social standing to intervene between my duty and my patient;

I will maintain the utmost respect for human life, from the time of conception; even under threat, I will not use my medical knowledge contrary to the laws of humanity.

I make these promises solemnly, freely and upon my honor.

INTERNATIONAL CODE OF NURSING ETHICS

Professional nurses minister to the sick, assume responsibility for creating a physical, social and spiritual environment which will be conducive to recovery, and stress the prevention of illness and promotion of health by teaching and example. They render health-service to the individual, the family, and the community and coordinate their services with members of other health professions.

Service to mankind is the primary function of nurses and the reason for the existence of the nursing profession. Need for nursing service is universal. Professional nursing service is therefore unrestricted by considerations of nationality, race, creed, colour, politics, or social status.

Inherent in the code is the fundamental concept that the nurse believes in the essential freedoms of mankind and in the preservation of human life.

The profession recognizes that an international code cannot cover in detail all the activities and relationships of nurses, some of which are conditioned by personal philosophies and beliefs.

Autonomy	Veracity	Nonmaleficence	Beneficence	Confidentiality	Justice	Rank

1. The fundamental responsibility of the nurse is threefold: to conserve life, to alleviate suffering, and to promote health.

Autonomy	Veracity	Nonmaleficence	Beneficence	Confidentiality	Justice	Rank

2. The nurse must maintain at all times the highest standards of nursing care and of professional conduct.

Autonomy	Veracity	Nonmaleficence	Beneficence	Confidentiality	Justice	Rank

3. The nurse must not only be well prepared to practice but must maintain her knowledge and skill at a consistently high level.

Autonomy	Veracity	Nonmaleficence	Beneficence	Confidentiality	Justice	Rank

	Autonomy	Veracity	Nonmaleficence	Beneficence	Confidentiality	Justice	Rank
4. The religious beliefs of a patient must be respected.							
5. Nurses hold in confidence all personal information entrusted to them.							
6. A nurse recognizes not only the responsibilities but the limitations of her or his professional functions; recommends or gives medical treatment without medical orders only in emergencies and reports such action to a physician at the earliest possible moment.							
7. The nurse is under an obligation to carry out the physician's orders intelligently and loyally and to refuse to participate in unethical procedures.							
8. The nurse sustains confidence in the physician and other members of the health team: incompetence or unethical conduct of associates should be exposed but only to the proper authority.							
9. A nurse is entitled to just remuneration and accepts only such compensation as the contract, actual or implied, provides.							
10. Nurses do not permit their names to be used in connection with the advertisement of products or with any other form of self-advertisement.							

Autonomy	Veracity	Nonmaleficence	Beneficence	Confidentiality	Justice	Rank

11. The nurse cooperates with and maintains harmonious relationships with members of other professions and with her or his nursing colleagues.

12. The nurse in private life adheres to standards of personal ethics which reflect credit upon her profession.

13. In personal conduct nurses should not knowingly disregard the accepted patterns of behaviour of the community in which they live and work.

14. A nurse should participate and share responsibility with other citizens and other health professions in promoting efforts to meet the health needs of the public—local, state, national and international.

THE NUREMBERG CODE

1. The voluntary consent of the human subject is *absolutely* essential.

   This means that the person involved should have legal capacity to give consent; should be so situated as to be able to exercise free power of choice, without the intervention of any element of force, fraud, deceit, duress, overreaching, or other ulterior form of constraint

Autonomy	Veracity	Nonmaleficence	Beneficence	Confidentiality	Justice	Rank

or coercion; and should have sufficient knowledge and comprehension of the elements of the subject matter involved as to enable him to make an understanding and enlightened decision. This latter element requires that before the acceptance of an affirmative decision by the experimental subject there should be made known to him the nature, duration, and purpose of the experiment; the method and means by which it is to be conducted; all inconveniences and hazards reasonably to be expected; and the effects upon his health or person which may possibly come from his participation in the experiment.

The duty and responsibility for ascertaining the quality of the consent rests upon each individual who initiates, directs, or engages in the experiment. It is a personal duty and responsibility which may not be delegated to another with impunity.

2. The experiment should be such as to yield fruitful results for the good of society, unprocurable by other methods or means of study, and not random and unnecessary in nature.

3. The experiment should be so designed and based on the results of

	Autonomy	Veracity	Nonmaleficence	Beneficence	Confidentiality	Justice	Rank

animal experimentation and a knowledge of the natural history of the disease or other problem under study that the anticipated results will justify the performance of the experiment.

4. The experiment should be so conducted as to avoid all unnecessary physical and mental suffering and injury.

5. No experiment should be conducted where there is an *a priori* reason to believe that death or disabling injury will occur; except, perhaps, in those experiments where the experimental physicians also serve as subjects.

6. The degree of risk to be taken should never exceed that determined by the humanitarian importance of the problem to be solved by the experiment.

7. Proper preparations should be made and adequate facilities provided to protect the experimental subject against even remote possibilities of injury, disability, or death.

8. The experiment should be conducted only by scientifically qualified persons. The highest degree of skill and care should be required through all stages of the experiment

Autonomy	Veracity	Nonmaleficence	Beneficence	Confidentiality	Justice	Rank

of those who conduct or engage in the experiment.

9. During the course of the experiment the human subject should be at liberty to bring the experiment to an end if he has reached the physical or mental state where continuation of the experiment seems to him to be impossible.

10. During the course of the experiment the scientist in charge must be prepared to terminate the experiment at any stage, if he has probable cause to believe, in the exercise of the good faith, superior skill, and careful judgment required of him that a continuation of the experiment is likely to result in injury, disability, or death to the experimental subject.

INTERNATIONAL CODE OF MEDICAL ETHICS

Adopted by the Third General Assembly of The World Medical Association, London, England, October 1949.

Duties of Doctors in General

A doctor must always maintain the highest standards of professional conduct.

	Autonomy	Veracity	Nonmaleficence	Beneficence	Confidentiality	Justice	Rank

A doctor must practice his profession uninfluenced by motives of profit.

The following practices are deemed unethical:

a) Any self advertisement except such as is expressly authorized by the national code of medical ethics.

b) Collaborate in any form of medical service in which the doctor does not have professional independence.

c) Receiving any money in connection with services rendered to a patient other than a proper professional fee, even with the knowledge of the patient.

Any act, or advice which could weaken physical or mental resistance of a human being may be used only in his interest.

A doctor is advised to use great caution in divulging discoveries or new techniques of treatment.

A doctor should certify or testify only to that which he has personally verified.

Duties of Doctors to the Sick

A doctor must always bear in mind the obligation of preserving human life.

Autonomy	Veracity	Nonmaleficence	Beneficence	Confidentiality	Justice	Rank

A doctor owes to his patient complete loyalty and all the resources of his science. Whenever an examination or treatment is beyond his capacity he should summon another doctor who has the necessary ability.

A doctor shall preserve absolute secrecy on all he knows about his patient because of the confidence entrusted in him.

A doctor must give emergency care as a humanitarian duty unless he is assured that others are willing and able to give such care.

Duties of Doctors to Each Other

A doctor ought to behave to his colleagues as he would have them behave to him.

A doctor must not entice patients from his colleagues.

A doctor must observe the principles of "The Declaration of Geneva" approved by The World Medical Association.

DECLARATION OF HELSINKI

Recommendations guiding medical doctors in biomedical research involving human subjects, adopted by the 18th World Medical Assembly, Helsinki, Finland, 1964, and revised by the 29th World Medical Assembly, Tokyo, Japan, 1975.

Autonomy	Veracity	Nonmaleficence	Beneficence	Confidentiality	Justice	Rank

Introduction

It is the mission of the medical doctor to safeguard the health of the people. His or her knowledge and conscience are dedicated to the fulfillment of this mission.

The Declaration of Geneva of the World Medical Association binds the doctor with the world, "The health of my patient will be my first consideration," and the International Code of Medical Ethics declares that, "Any act or advice which could weaken physical or mental resistance of a human being may be used only in his interest."

The purpose of biomedical research involving human subjects must be to improve diagnostic, therapeutic and prophylactic procedures and the understanding of the aetiology and pathogenesis of disease.

In current medical practice most diagnostic, therapeutic or prophylactic procedures involve hazards. This applies *a fortiori* to biomedical research.

Medical progress is based on research which ultimately must rest in part on experimentation involving human subjects.

Autonomy	Veracity	Nonmaleficence	Beneficence	Confidentiality	Justice	Rank

In the field of biomedical research a fundamental distinction must be recognized between medical research in which the aim is essentially diagnostic or therapeutic for a patient, and medical research, the essential object of which is purely scientific and without direct diagnostic or therapeutic value to the person subjected to the research.

Special caution must be exercised in the conduct of research which may affect the environment, and the welfare of animals used for research must be respected.

Because it is essential that the results of laboratory experiments be applied to human beings to further scientific knowledge and to help suffering humanity, The World Medical Association has prepared the following recommendations as a guide to every doctor in biomedical research involving human subjects. They should be kept under review in the future. It must be stressed that the standards as drafted are only a guide to physicians all over the world. Doctors are not relieved from criminal, civil and ethical responsibilities under the laws of their own countries.

I. Basic Principles

1. Biomedical research involving human subjects must conform to gen-

Autonomy	Veracity	Nonmaleficence	Beneficence	Confidentiality	Justice	Rank

erally accepted scientific principles and should be based on adequately performed laboratory and animal experimentation and on a thorough knowledge of the scientific literature.

2. The design and performance of each experimental procedure involving human subjects should be clearly formulated in an experimental protocol which should be transmitted to a specially appointed independent committee for consideration, comment and guidance.

3. Biomedical research involving human subjects should be conducted only by scientifically qualified persons and under the supervision of a clinically competent medical person. The responsibility for the human subject must always rest with a medically qualified person and never rest on the subject of the research, even though the subject has given his or her consent.

4. Biomedical research involving human subjects cannot legitimately be carried out unless the importance of the objective is in proportion to the inherent risk to the subject.

5. Every biomedical research project involving human subjects should be

Autonomy	Veracity	Nonmaleficence	Beneficence	Confidentiality	Justice	Rank

preceded by careful assessment of predictable risks in comparison with forseeable benefits to the subject or to others. Concern for the interests of the subject must always prevail over the interest of science and society.

6. The right of the research subject to safeguard his or her integrity must always be respected. Every precaution should be taken to respect the privacy of the subject and to minimize the impact of the study on the subject's physical and mental integrity and on the personality of the subject.

7. Doctors should abstain from engaging in research projects involving human subjects unless they are satisfied that the hazards involved are believed to be predictable. Doctors should cease any investigation if the hazards are found to outweigh the potential benefits.

8. In publication of the results of his or her research, the doctor is obliged to preserve the accuracy of the results. Reports of experimentation not in accordance with the principles laid down in this Declaration should not be accepted for publication.

Autonomy	Veracity	Nonmaleficence	Beneficence	Confidentiality	Justice	Rank

9. In any research on human beings, each potential subject must be adequately informed of the aims, methods, anticipated benefits and potential hazards of the study and the discomfort it may entail. He or she should be informed that he or she is at liberty to abstain from participation in the study and that he or she is free to withdraw his or her consent to participation at any time. The doctor should then obtain the subject's freely given informed consent, preferably in writing.

10. When obtaining informed consent for the research project the doctor should be particularly cautious if the subject is in a dependent relationship to him or her or may consent under duress. In that case the informed consent should be obtained by a doctor who is not engaged in the investigation and who is completely independent of this official relationship.

11. In case of legal incompetence, informed consent should be obtained from the legal guardian in accordance with national legislation. Where physical or mental incapacity makes it impossible to obtain informed consent, or when the subject is a minor, permission from the respon-

	Autonomy	Veracity	Nonmaleficence	Beneficence	Confidentiality	Justice	Rank

sible relative replaces that of the subject in accordance with national legislation.

12. The research protocol should always contain a statement of the ethical considerations involved and should indicate that the principles enunciated in the present Declaration are complied with.

II. Medical Research Combined with Professional Care (Clinical Research)

1. In the treatment of the sick person, the doctor must be free to use a new diagnostic and therapeutic measure, if in his or her judgment it offers hope of saving life, reestablishing health or alleviating suffering.

2. The potential benefits, hazards and discomfort of a new method should be weighed against the advantages of the best current diagnostic and therapeutic methods.

3. In any medical study, every patient—including those of a control group, if any—should be assured of the best proven diagnostic and therapeutic method.

4. The refusal of the patient to participate in a study must never interfere with the doctor-patient relationship.

Autonomy	Veracity	Nonmaleficence	Beneficence	Confidentiality	Justice	Rank

5. If the doctor considers it essential not to obtain informed consent, the specific reasons for this proposal should be stated in the experimental protocol for transmission to the independent committee (I,2).

6. The doctor can combine medical research with professional care, the objective being the acquisition of new medical knowledge, only to the extent that medical research is justified by its potential diagnostic or therapeutic value for the patient.

III. Non-therapeutic Biomedical Research Involving Human Subjects (Non-clinical Biomedical Research)

1. In the purely scientific application of medical research carried out on a human being, it is the duty of the doctor to remain the protector of the life and health of that person on whom biomedical research is being carried out.

2. The subjects should be volunteers—either healthy persons or patients for whom the experimental design is not related to the patient's illness.

3. The investigator or the investigating team should discontinue the research if in his/her or their judgment

Autonomy	Veracity	Nonmaleficence	Beneficence	Confidentiality	Justice	Rank

it may, if continued, be harmful to the individual.

4. In research on man, the interest of science and society should never take precedence over considerations related to the well being of the subject.

AMERICAN MEDICAL ASSOCIATION ETHICAL GUIDELINES FOR CLINICAL INVESTIGATION

The following guidelines are intended to aid physicians in fulfilling their ethical responsibilities when they engage in the clinical investigation of new drugs and procedures.

(1) A physician may participate in clinical investigation only to the extent that those activities are a part of a systematic program competently designed, under accepted standards of scientific research, to produce data which is scientifically valid and significant.

(2) In conducting clinical investigation, the investigator should demonstrate the same concern and caution for the welfare, safety, and comfort of the person involved as is required of a physician who is furnishing medical

Autonomy	Veracity	Nonmaleficence	Beneficence	Confidentiality	Justice	Rank

care to a patient independent of any clinical investigation.

(3) In clinical investigation primarily for treatment—

A. The physician must recognize that the physician-patient relationship exists and that professional judgment and skill must be exercised in the best interest of the patient.

B. Voluntary written consent must be obtained from the patient, or from his legally authorized representative if the patient lacks the capacity to consent, following: (a) disclosure that the physician intends to use an investigational drug or experimental procedure, (b) a reasonable explanation of the nature of the drug or procedure to be used, risks to be expected, and possible therapeutic benefits, (c) an offer to answer any inquiries concerning the drug or procedure, and (d) a disclosure of alternative drugs or procedures that may be available.

i. In exceptional circumstances and to the extent that disclosure of information concerning the nature of the drug or experimental procedure or risks would be expected to

Autonomy	Veracity	Nonmaleficence	Beneficence	Confidentiality	Justice	Rank

materially affect the health of the patient and would be detrimental to his best interests, such information may be withheld from the patient. In such circumstances, such information shall be disclosed to a responsible relative or friend of the patient where possible.

ii. Ordinarily, consent should be in writing, except where the physician deems it necessary to rely upon consent in other than written form because of the physical or emotional state of the patient.

iii. Where emergency treatment is necessary, the patient is incapable of giving consent, and no one is available who has authority to act on his behalf; consent is assumed.

(4) In clinical investigation primarily for the accumulation of scientific knowledge—
A. Adequate safeguards must be provided for the welfare, safety and comfort of the subject. It is fundamental social policy that the advancement of scientific knowledge must always be secondary to primary concern for the individual.

Autonomy	Veracity	Nonmaleficence	Beneficence	Confidentiality	Justice	Rank

B. Consent, in writing, should be obtained from the subject, or from his legally authorized representative if the subject lacks the capacity to consent, following: (a) a disclosure of the fact that an investigational drug or procedure is to be used, (b) a reasonable explanation of the nature of the procedure to be used and risks to be expected, and (c) an offer to answer any inquiries concerning the drug or procedure.

C. Minors or mentally incompetent persons may be used as subjects only if:

   i. The nature of the investigation is such that mentally competent adults would not be suitable subjects.

   ii. Consent, in writing, is given by a legally authorized representative of the subject under circumstances in which an informed and prudent adult would reasonably be expected to volunteer himself or his child as a subject.

D. No person may be used as a subject against his will.

E. The overuse of institutionalized persons in research is an unfair

Autonomy	Veracity	Nonmaleficence	Beneficence	Confidentiality	Justice	Rank

distribution of research risks. Participation is coercive and not voluntary if the participant is subjected to powerful incentives and persuasion.

(*Current Opinions of the Judicial Council of the AMA*, 1982. Reprinted with permission of the American Medical Association.)

AMERICAN MEDICAL TECHNOLOGISTS CODE OF ETHICS

Recognizing that the American Medical Technologists seeks to encourage, establish and maintain the highest standards, traditions, and principles of our profession as a condition of Registration and maintaining membership in good standing in the American Medical Technologists, I pledge myself to practice Medical Technology in strict accord with the principles, standards, traditions and regulations of the American Medical Technologists and in accordance with the laws of the state in which I practice.

While engaged in the Arts and Sciences which constitute the practice of Medical Technology, I shall practice with thorough self-restraint, always placing the welfare of the patients, entrusted to my care for tests or examinations, above all else, with full realization of my per-

Autonomy	Veracity	Nonmaleficence	Beneficence	Confidentiality	Justice	Rank

sonal responsibility for the patients' best interests.

Realizing that it is incumbent upon me, as a Medical Technologist to continually keep abreast of the times, I pledge myself to strive constantly to increase my technical knowledge of Medical Technology and to participate in the interchange of knowledge with other competent practitioners of Medical Technology and or other paramedical Arts and Sciences that our joint knowledge shall benefit the profession and my practice.

I pledge accuracy and reliability in the performance of tests and to seek competent professional council when in doubt of my own judgment or competence in a particular test or examination.

As a further consideration for registration, I pledge myself to avoid dishonest, unethical or illegal compensation for such services as I shall render to the patients in my charge and I shall shun unwarranted professional publicity or unjust discrimination among the patients in my charge.

I pledge myself to protect the judgment of the attending physician in all cases in which I am directed to make laboratory tests or examinations, and to report the results of my findings free

Autonomy	Veracity	Nonmaleficence	Beneficence	Confidentiality	Justice	Rank

from all personal opinion to the attending physician only. I shall not make or offer a diagnosis or interpretation unless I be a duly licensed physician, except as the results of the report may of itself so indicate, or unless I am asked to by the attending physician.

I pledge myself to protect the identity and the integrity of all patients placed in my charge and to make only such reports public as shall be required by me by the laws of the state in which I practice or as the patient's physician shall direct.

As a final condition of Registration and Membership in the American Medical Technologists, I pledge my honor and my integrity to cooperate in the advancement and expansion, by every lawful means within my power, of the influence of the American Medical Technologists and to defend its principles.

(Reprinted with permission of the American Medical Technologists Association.)

AMERICAN SOCIETY OF RADIOLOGIC TECHNOLOGISTS CODE OF ETHICS

Preamble. This Code of Ethics is to serve as a guide by which Radiologic Technologists may evaluate their profes-

Autonomy	Veracity	Nonmaleficence	Beneficence	Confidentiality	Justice	Rank

sional conduct as it relates to patients, colleagues, other members of the allied professions and health care consumers.

The Code of Ethics is not law but is intended to assist Radiologic Technologists in maintaining a high level of ethical conduct.

Therefore, in the practice of the profession, we the members of the American Society of Radiologic Technologists, accept the following principles:

Principle 1. Radiologic Technologists shall conduct themselves in a manner compatible with the dignity of their profession.

Principle 2. Radiologic Technologists shall provide services with consideration of human dignity and the uniqueness of the patient, unrestricted by considerations of age, sex, race, creed, social or economic status, handicap, personal attributes or the nature of the health problem.

Principle 3. Radiologic Technologists shall make every effort to protect all patients from unnecessary radiation.

Principle 4. Radiologic Technologists should exercise and accept responsibility for independent discretion and judgement in the performance of their professional services.

Principle 5. Radiologic Technologists shall judiciously protect the patient's right to privacy and shall maintain all patient information in the strictest confidence.

Principle 6. Radiologic Technologists shall apply only methods of technology

Autonomy	Veracity	Nonmaleficence	Beneficence	Confidentiality	Justice	Rank

founded upon a scientific basis and not accept those methods that violate this principle.

Principle 7. Radiologic Technologists shall not diagnose, but in recognition of their responsibility to the patient, they shall provide the physician with all information they have relative to radiologic diagnosis or patient management.

Principle 8. Radiologic Technologists shall be responsible for reporting unethical conduct and illegal professional activities to the appropriate authorities.

Principle 9. Radiologic Technologists should continually strive to improve their knowledge and skills by participating in educational and professional activities and sharing the benefits of their attainments with their colleagues.

Principle 10. Radiologic Technologists should protect the public from misinformation and misrepresentations.

(Reprinted with permission of the American Society of Radiologic Technologists.)

CODE OF ETHICS OF THE AMERICAN ASSOCIATION FOR RESPIRATORY THERAPY

As Allied Health professionals engaged in the performance of Respiratory Ther-

Autonomy	Veracity	Nonmaleficence	Beneficence	Confidentiality	Justice	Rank

apy, we realize we must individually and collectively strive to maintain the highest obtainable level of ethical standards.

The principles set forth define the ethical and moral standards to which each member of the American Association for Respiratory Therapy should conform. This Code of Ethics shall be subject to monitoring, interpretation, and timely revision by the Association's Board of Directors, with the advice of the Board of Medical Advisors.

Each member of this Association shall conduct himself in such a manner as to gain the respect and confidence of other Health Care personnel, as well as respecting the human dignity of each of his superiors, subordinates, and other associates.

Each member shall be responsible for the competent and efficient execution of his assigned duties, being guided at all times by his concern for the welfare of the patient.

Each member shall be familiar with, and comply with existing state and/or federal laws governing the practice of Respiratory Therapy.

Each member shall keep in confidence any and all privileged information concerning the patient. Inquiries

Autonomy	Veracity	Nonmaleficence	Beneficence	Confidentiality	Justice	Rank

regarding the dissemination of privileged personal or clinical information pertaining to the patient by persons other than those members of the Health Care team who are responsible for the care of the patient, shall be referred to the physician in charge of the patient's medical care.

No member shall endeavor to extend his province beyond his competence and the authority invested to him by a physician.

No member shall accept gratuities in the form of bribes or tips for preferential consideration of the patient, or to supplement professional income. The member must carefully guard against conflicts of professional interest.

Each member shall accept responsibility for exposing incompetence and illegal or unethical conduct to the proper authorities and/or the Judicial Committee of this Association. Only through the integrity of each member can the highest purpose of the profession be served.

Each member shall adhere to the Bylaws of the Association and support the objectives and purposes contained therein.

(Reprinted with permission of the American Association for Respiratory Therapy.)

CODE OF ETHICS FOR THE AMERICAN PHYSICAL THERAPY ASSOCIATION

Adopted by APTA House of Delegates, June 1978.

Preamble. The physical therapist member of the American Physical Therapy Association accepts this Code of Ethics as the basis for the practice of his profession. Individually and collectively, these members of the Association are responsible for promoting and maintaining the highest ethical standards.

There shall always be a Guide for Professional Conduct to assist in the interpretation of the Code of Ethics. This guide, taking reference from the code, shall be subject to monitoring and timely revision by the Association's Judicial Committee.

This Code of Ethics and the Guide for Professional Conduct shall be binding on the physical therapist members.

Principle 1. The physical therapist should respect the dignity of each individual with whom he is associated in the practice of his profession.

Principle 2. The physical therapist should comply with the law and Association policies governing the practice of physical therapy.

Principle 3. The physical therapist should accept responsibility for the exercise of professional judgment.

Principle 4. The physical therapist should maintain optimal standards of professional practice.

Autonomy	Veracity	Nonmaleficence	Beneficence	Confidentiality	Justice	Rank

	Autonomy	Veracity	Nonmaleficence	Beneficence	Confidentiality	Justice	Rank

Principle 5. The physical therapist should respect the confidences imparted to him in the course of his professional activities.

Principle 6. The physical therapist should seek reasonable, deserved, and fiscally sound remuneration for his services.

Principle 7. The physical therapist should provide accurate information to the consumer about the profession and services provided by the individual physical therapist.

Principle 8. The physical therapist should accept responsibility for reporting alleged incompetence, illegal activities, and/or unethical conduct to the proper authority.

Principle 9. The physical therapist should so conduct himself in all of his affairs as to avoid discredit to the Association and to the profession.

Principle 10. The physical therapist should give his loyalty and support to the American Physical Therapy Association in its efforts to attain its objectives.

(Reprinted with permission of the American Physical Therapy Association.)

Autonomy	Veracity	Nonmaleficence	Beneficence	Confidentiality	Justice	Rank

CODE FOR NURSES

Adopted by the American Nurses' Association

1. The nurse provides services with respect for human dignity and the uniqueness of the client unrestricted by considerations of social or economic status, personal attributes, or the nature of health problems.

2. The nurse safeguards the client's right to privacy by judiciously protecting information of a confidential nature.

3. The nurse acts to safeguard the client and the public when health care and safety are affected by the incompetent, unethical, or illegal practice of any person.

4. The nurse assumes responsibility and accountability for individual nursing judgments and actions.

5. The nurse maintains competence in nursing.

6. The nurse exercises informed judgment and uses individual competence and qualifications as criteria in seeking consultation, accepting responsibilities, and delegating nursing activities to others.

	Autonomy	Veracity	Nonmaleficence	Beneficence	Confidentiality	Justice	Rank

7. The nurse participates in activities that contribute to the ongoing development of the profession's body of knowledge.

8. The nurse participates in the profession's efforts to implement and improve standards of nursing.

9. The nurse participates in the profession's efforts to establish and maintain conditions of employment conducive to high quality nursing care.

10. The nurse participates in the profession's efforts to protect the public from misinformation and misrepresentation and maintain the integrity of nursing.

11. The nurse collaborates with members of the health professions and other citizens in promoting community and national efforts to meet the health needs of the public.

After you rank each guideline for its ethical importance on a scale of 1 for minimal value and 5 for very important (in the last box of each line), outline your thoughts or guidelines that should be added to the professional code.

4 IDENTIFYING AND WEIGHTING ETHICAL RULES

CHAPTER 4 EXERCISE
IDENTIFYING AND WEIGHTING
ETHICAL RULES

NAME

CLASS

Phase One

Where did you fall on the conservative–liberal spectrum with the six statements about distributive justice given in the first part of Chapter 4? Check your score below:

Very liberal			Moderate			Very conservative
6	10	14	18	22	26	30

How does this evaluation agree with your own self-evaluation? How does it agree with your world view as examined in Chapter 1? If your are conservative you should be more inclined to the fixed philosophy of nature; if you are liberal, then you should be inclined toward the process world view. Do you see any relationship between your conservative or liberal perspective of these six issues of justice and the male/female approach to ethical dilemmas outlined by Piaget, Kohlberg, and Gilligan? Comment in the space below and on the next page.

_____

_____

_____

_____

_____

_____

Phase Two

In the space below and on the next page create a list of ethical rules or guidelines derived from the principle of justice as related to the employment of health professionals. The case below will give you a focus. Your statements can include such phrases as: "Health professionals should (have a right to) . . ." and "Health professionals are responsible for (should be allowed to, have a right to, should never). . . ."

On August 4, a student finishing up the clinical portion of an allied health training program was interviewed for a position at a nearby hospital. Although not scheduled to graduate for another month, the student had passed the registry examination. The student was offered the position, accepted it, and agreed to commence employment on Tuesday, September 28, at 9:00 AM.

In the 55-day interval between the initial interview on August 4 and September 28, the physician and the supervising allied health professional at the hospital spoke with the student three times on the telephone and had a second in-person meeting. In all four conversations, the student appeared enthusiastic about being employed at the hospital and eager to begin. Although the supervising allied health professional required immediate assistance, he was willing to wait until the student was available. The hospital considered the position filled and dissuaded other qualified candidates.

On the morning of September 28, the student called at 8:55 and stated that he would not report for work unless the hospital would match in salary and benefits a job offer the student had received a few days earlier. The physician informed the student the hospital would not reconsider its employment agreement and considered this demand inconsiderate, unfair to the staff and patients at the hospital, dishonorable, and unprofessional. The physician informed the student's allied health dean, the clinical supervisors, and the college personnel office of the student's action.

In the space below and on the next page list guidelines and rules related to the principle of justice that apply to this case. Keep in mind the rights and responsibilities of the health professional being employed, the hospital employing the student, and the consequences of the student's action for the hospital staff and patients.

_____
_____
_____
_____
_____
_____
_____
_____
_____
_____
_____
_____
_____
_____
_____
_____
_____
_____
_____
_____
_____
_____
_____
_____
_____
_____
_____
_____

Phase Three

Select from your list of guidelines in Phase Two six to 10 values at random or those that are more important to you. Rank these below with the most important guideline at the top and the least important at the bottom. Give each statement an order number depending on its relative importance in this list, with 10 being most important and 1 being least important (see directions on page 56).

Add up your order numbers to get your total. Enter this total at the bottom of the list.

Calculate the weighting factor for each of your guidelines. Divide the order number by the total to get each weighting factor.

	Order	Weighting Factor
1.		
2.		
3.		
4.		
5.		
6.		
7.		
8.		

Order	Weighting Factor

9. _____

_____

_____

10. _____

_____

_____

Total =

Outline your thoughts in rough form here before composing your final answers for this exercise.

5   MAKING TRIAGE DECISIONS

CHAPTER 5 EXERCISE
MAKING TRIAGE DECISIONS

NAME

CLASS

Phase One

The following situation is totally unrealistic and could not occur in a real health care situation, but it provides a useful frame for practicing and understanding triage decisions.

One Monday morning you arrive at the hospital where you are in clinical training as a physical therapist. You are just in time for your first participation in the Ethics and Resources Committee meeting. As you approach the conference room, you find it strangely quiet. No one is around. On the conference table are telephone messages from the social worker, the chaplains, the rehabilitation specialist, the consumer representatives, and everyone else on the committee, reporting their inability to be at the meeting. You are the only member of the committee present.

There is also a folder with a note from the Medical Director who is out with the flu. Reading the note, you learn that the committee must make a decision within the hour on the use of the two Hubbard (antibiotic) baths in the intensive care burn unit.

There was a terrible four-alarm apartment fire in the city on Sunday. As a result, eight patients were admitted who require extensive treatment utilizing the Hubbard baths. Pulling out the patient records, you find the following information about the candidates:

1. Male, age 57, politician, gay, divorced, no dependents

2. Female child, age 3

3. Male, age 63, army general, married, seven children

4. Female, age 28, government worker, Nobel prize nominee, single

5. Male, age 30, teacher, just married, no children

6. Female, about 50, other details unknown

7. Male, age 60, Vietnamese immigrant, widowed, no family

8. Teenager, gender not indicated on admissions form.

Medical opinion is that each of the burn patients has an equal chance of survival and recovery if given regular treatment with the Hubbard bath. Each patient has third degree burns over 50–60% of the body. As the physical therapist, you will be responsible for debridement of the burned areas and assisting while the bandages are peeled off three times a day prior to immersion of the patient in the antibiotic saline solution of the Hubbard bath. Without this thrice daily treatment, the patient will die of massive infections and fluid loss that cannot be controlled with intravenous saline.

Only four patients can be treated successfully, two on each of the Hubbard facilities. Because of a blizzard, it is impossible to transfer any of the patients to another hospital. Which four do you select for treatment? Circle your four choices.

1. Male politician

2. Female child

3. Army general

4. Female government worker

5. Male school teacher

6. Unidentified female

7. Vietnamese male

8. Teenager

What are your reasons for your four choices?

_____

_____

_____

_____

_____

_____

_____

_____

While you are pondering your choices and wonder whether you have made the right decisions, the medical records department sends up more information on the eight patients.

Patient 1:   A male politician, age 57. You recognize his name from recent headlines in the newspapers. There has been considerable controversy and some scandal over his shady connections and allegations of kickback schemes since hundreds of thousands of dollars have been unaccountably deposited in his bank accounts. He has denied any illegal activity, but several close associates are now serving time in federal prisons after conviction on various charges. The District Attorney's office has said there is insufficient evidence to justify a grand jury investigation. The man has also been involved in several alimony cases with his four ex-wives. He is currently living with a male lover and has no minor children to support.

Patient 2:   A female child, age 3. She also is familiar to you from the newspapers. Her picture was on the front page as the "miracle baby." Her parents tried for 17 years to have a child. Finally, the couple had been accepted for treatment at the new embryo transplant facility in western Virginia. The new technique worked and the woman became pregnant after test tube fertilization and implantation of the embryo.

Patient 3:   An army general, age 63. Veteran of many campaigns in Vietnam and Cambodia, the general had ordered the aerial spraying of Agent Orange defoliant, which has recently brought countless law suits from veterans claiming serious health problems from their exposure to it. Mixing a military career with married life, the general has seven children, all under age 18 and all showing great promise of contributing to the good of society.

Patient 4:   A female government worker, age 28. The first Mexican-American woman appointed to head the federal Department of Health and Welfare, she is a nominee for the Nobel Peace Prize this year because of her championing of the rights of millions of refugees from political anarchy, civil wars, droughts, and famine around the world. She gained fame for her successful personal persuasion of the heads of states in the developed nations to establish a unified global refugee and foreign aid program. She has never married.

Patient 5:   A male high school teacher, age 30. Just married, he has no children. However, he is the sole support of his widowed mother, age 68, who is a bed-ridden invalid.

Patient 6:   An unidentified female of unknown background. Apparently about 50, she was found severely burned in the basement, behind the boiler, where she appears to have been living for some time when not begging on the streets. She is what the social worker would call a ''bag lady,'' with no home or known relatives. Several bank pass books in her shopping bag indicate she is actually very wealthy.

Patient 7:   A Vietnamese male, about 60 years old. A window washer and general maintenance man in the apartment, he had been a very successful medical researcher and social leader in his own country before the Communists forced his exile. In this country, he has spent most of his spare time helping set up informal schools to teach citizenship and English to political refugees from Southeast Asia. Widowed with no immediate family.

Patient 8:   A teenager by the name of Kelly. For some reason, the file on this patient leaves the teenager's sex unlisted. The file has only medical notations with nothing about the patient's background. The patient has not been rational enough to provide any information though he or she has been informed that the rest of the family perished in the fire.

Reevaluate your original choices. Have you changed your choices? If so, what new information prompted you to change?

_____

_____

_____

_____

_____

_____

_____

_____

_____

_____

_____

_____

_____

_____

Now in a second *déjà vu* of your one-person Ethics and Resources Committee, we find that the Medical Director is quite sensitive to the problems of triage decisions so, instead of eight medical files on the candidates, you find on the conference table only eight small index cards. On each card is a first name, as follows:

Card 1: Chris	Card 3: Robin	Card 5: Jamie	Card 7: Kelly
Card 2: Pat	Card 4: Tony	Card 6: Nicki	Card 8: Randy

Now, with only the eight names to go on, whom do you select? All information, relevant and irrelevant, has been eliminated. You cannot even be certain of the gender of the patients. You have no idea whether they are atheists or religious, married or single, homosexual or heterosexual, young, middle-aged, or old, with a family or alone. You also have no idea of their profession or occupation. Your only solution is to use a random lottery. Shuffle the index cards, and have someone pull the first four who will be treated.

A common experience with the foregoing exercise is that the more information given on the candidates, the more the decision becomes bogged down in often irrelevant criteria. Military people and politicians, especially if they are male, are quickly eliminated. The bias against older single persons is not as strong, but it is there. This bias might be reversed in a country like China where older people are highly respected. There are definite biases against homosexual persons, "socially useless" persons like vagrants, "bag women," drug addicts, "hippy" teenagers, and against "dangerous" people like atheists, communists, and radicals of any kind.

How did you fare in the first two situations when you had a fair amount of information? What criteria, if any, did you select? Are these, in hindsight, morally relevant criteria?

_____

_____

_____

_____

_____

_____

_____

_____

Phase Two: Population Planning and Triage in the Philippines

In the Philippines, where families with eight or 10 children are common, the Government, Roman Catholic Church leaders, international monetary funds, and the developed nations clashed head-on in mid-1982. It started on July 6, 1982, when Prime Minister César Virata announced that steps must be taken immediately to prevent the Philippine population, then at 50 million, from more than doubling in the subsequent 30 years. This doubling, only three decades off at the present annual growth rate of 2.5%, would bring the island nation close to the limits of its resources. Some experts see the Philippines as another India and Manila as a rival of Calcutta if this trend continues.*

Having just returned from a meeting of the World Bank in Tokyo, the Prime Minister told the Philippine Cabinet that prospects for increased financial assistance from other nations and from multilateral institutions such as the World Bank were very dim unless the country could bring its growth rate down and increase the use of contraceptives significantly. A few years ago the government set a goal of reducing the annual growth rate from 2.5% to 2% by 1985. Another goal set by the government was to increase contraceptive use from its present 39% to 83.5%, also by 1985. In mid-1982, neither goal was feasible. As a consequence, the government has very limited resources, clearly inadequate to create the 700,000 new jobs that will be needed each year to meet the demands of the growing workforce.

Although the use of contraceptives is far below economically desirable levels and the government's stated goals, more Catholics seem willing to ignore the official Church condemnation of contraception as sinful. Another trend, even more disturbing to Church leaders, is the growing acceptance of abortion. One survey indicates that one third of Philippine women and half of the health professionals believe abortion should be legalized under certain circumstances.

Church officials argue that overpopulation is largely an urban problem and can be solved by redistributing industry and labor opportunities equally between the villages and larger cities. The three million people in Manila, half of them destitute squatters, are expected to grow to over 12 million before the year 2000 unless something drastic is done. Church leaders strongly condemn any program based on advocacy of contraception and schedule regular sermons in all the churches on the sanctity of life and the blessings of motherhood.

Led by Economic Planning Director Placido Mapa, a member of a conservative religious order for laypersons, the Church won a temporary victory in May,

---

*This account is based on a press release from *The New York Times,* July 18, 1982, p. 8.

1982, by forcing the deletion of the family planning program from a draft of economic priorities for 1983 to 1987. However, a few months later, the government won Cabinet approval of an economic aid package from the United States. The sole purpose of this multimillion dollar assistance program is to help control population growth through education programs and distribution of free contraceptives.

With the current thinking on "lifeboat ethics," triage, and the overpopulation crisis in the Third World nations, it is not difficult to forecast some likely developments. In the not too distant future, multilateral institutions, like the World Bank and European Development Fund, and some of the rich developed nations may begin to put conditions on their shipments of food and their financial aid to the overpopulated developing nations like the Philippines. If the country is not making what is judged to be adequate efforts and progress in controlling its population growth, food, financial aid, and technological assistance will simply be denied. The overpopulated nations will be left to shift for themselves, like leaky, overcrowded lifeboats.

The argument may be made that providing surplus food, rich in protein, to starving people only increases their fertility. At the least, it reduces the death rate and thus indirectly contributes to the skyrocketing population problem. Some may argue that providing food to starving people may sound like the moral thing to do in the short run, but in the long run it only makes matters far worse by increasing the potential mass starvation if they have no effective population program.

What are your thoughts about this prospect? Is it ethical for a rich nation to make its financial assistance to developing nations dependent on those governments' ability to enforce the population control programs necessary for survival not just of these nations but also of the world? If you believe it is ethical, under what circumstances? What points can you find in the chapter to support your position? What ethical principles and values are involved in this case? Use one or two extra pages for your full discussion of this problem. Staple it to these exercise pages.

6 ANALYZING THE HEALTH CARE SOCIAL CONTRACT

CHAPTER 6 EXERCISE
ANALYZING THE HEALTH CARE
SOCIAL CONTRACT

NAME

CLASS

Phase One

In this section you have space to spell out the details of the implied contract patients commonly enter into with their health care professionals. In some questions it may be practical to divide your answer into two columns, one covering the patient viewpoint and the other applying to the health worker. With other questions, it may be easier to integrate the patient and health worker aspects in one or two statements.

1. Describe the nature and character of the "human relationship" as it should ideally exist between the patient and the health worker.

Patient   *Health Care Worker*

_____

_____

_____

_____

_____

_____

_____

_____

261

2. What obligations are accepted by the patient? By the health care worker?

Patient   *Health Care Worker*

_____   _____

_____   _____

_____   _____

_____   _____

_____   _____

3. What benefits can the patient expect from this contractual relationship? What benefits can the health worker expect? (A patient obligation may involve a benefit for the health worker and vice versa.)

Patient   *Health Care Worker*

_____   _____

_____   _____

_____   _____

_____   _____

_____   _____

4. How are decisions handled?
   a. In emergency situations?

Patient   *Health Care Worker*

_____   _____

_____   _____

_____   _____

_____   _____

_____   _____

b. In nonemergency or routine situations?

Patient   *Health Care Worker*

_____

_____

_____

_____

_____

c. In major decisions about treatment plan?

Patient   *Health Care Worker*

_____

_____

_____

_____

_____

5. How is the contract (relationship) terminated? Who can terminate it and under what circumstances?

Patient   *Health Care Worker*

_____

_____

_____

_____

_____

_____

_____

6. How are conflicts in the values of the health worker and the patient handled?

Patient   *Health Care Worker*

_____

_____

_____

_____

_____

_____

_____

benefit for the health worker and vice versa.)

Phase Two

Below are eight sets of conflicting rights and values. The first set is the essence of our earlier discussion of the conservative/liberal bias, the conflict between individual freedom and social responsibility. The others represent different levels of conflicting goals, values, or rules. Your task is the same as in the chapter. Consider each set separately and circle where you feel the compromise should be made. If you circle a 1 or a 10 for any set, you are indicating that the other value or rule has no real merit.*

Individual freedom   **Social responsibility**
1   2   3   4   5   6   7   8   9   10

Long, routine life   **Short, exciting life**
1   2   3   4   5   6   7   8   9   10

Parental rights   **Child's rights**
1   2   3   4   5   6   7   8   9   10

Rights of pregnant woman   **Rights of fetus under five months**
1   2   3   4   5   6   7   8   9   10

*This resolution of conflict exercise was suggested by Marion Kayhart, Cedar Crest College, Allentown, Pennsylvania, and by E. James Kennedy, North Park College, Chicago, Illinois.

Reasonable quality of life							Sanctity of human life itself		
1	2	3	4	5	6	7	8	9	10

Rights of children in family							Rights of unborn fetus		
1	2	3	4	5	6	7	8	9	10

							Obligation to genetic		
Right to have one's own children							health of future generations		
1	2	3	4	5	6	7	8	9	10

							Right not to be born with a		
Right to life of any fetus							serious crippling defect		
1	2	3	4	5	6	7	8	9	10

You may want to repeat this balancing of conflicts when you finish the course to see whether your values and views have shifted, and if so, in what direction.

Phase Three

It is not uncommon for a patient to confide in a therapist, nurse, technician, or clinician information that he or she has not shared with the physician in charge of the case. When it is important that the physician be aware of this information, a conflict of values may arise if the patient explicitly forbids the passing on of this information by the health care worker to the physician. What are your thoughts on how this conflict between the patient's good and the obligation of confidentiality might be resolved?

_____

_____

_____

_____

_____

_____

_____

_____

_____

Check the professional codes in the Chapter 3 Exercise. Does your professional code, or those of other professions, give any guidelines for resolving the conflicting obligations of confidentiality, autonomy, and truth telling? If nothing is stated in your professional code, are you aware of any informal policy on this matter? Ask someone already working in the clinical setting, your program director, clinical faculty, or medical director about this. Briefly summarize what you discover.

_____

_____

_____

_____

_____

_____

_____

_____

_____

_____

_____

_____

_____

_____

_____

_____

_____

_____

_____

_____

_____

Outline your thoughts in rough form here before composing your final answers for this exercise.

CHAPTER 7 EXERCISE
IDENTIFYING AND SORTING ALTERNATIVES

CASE TITLE

NAME

CLASS

Warm-up and Review

Identify and list by number the specific ethical issues, concerns, and principles involved in this case.

YOUR LIST OF ETHICAL ISSUES

1. _____

_____

2. _____

_____

3. _____

_____

4. _____

_____

5. _____

_____

6. _____

_____

7. _____

_____

8. _____

_____

9. _____

_____

10. _____

_____

11. _____

_____

12. _____

_____

13. _____

_____

14. _____

_____

Phase One

List below as many options as you can for this case.

	Professional Code	Personal Values	Value Optimizing	Interest Group

YOUR LIST OF ALTERNATIVES

1. _____

_____

2. _____

_____

3. _____

_____

4. _____

_____

Professional Code	Personal Values	Value Optimizing	Interest Group

5. _____

_____

6. _____

_____

7. _____

_____

8. _____

_____

9. _____

_____

10. _____

_____

11. _____

_____

12. _____

_____

13. _____

_____

14. _____

_____

15. _____

_____

16. _____

_____

	Professional Code	Personal Values	Value Optimizing	Interest Group

17. _____

_____

18. _____

_____

19. _____

_____

20. _____

_____

21. _____

_____

22. _____

_____

23. _____

_____

24. _____

_____

25. _____

_____

Phase Two

Put an X in the first box after any alternative that violates an ethical principle or guideline in your *professional code*. Then put an X in the second box after any alternative that violates your own *personal ethical principles*. Then cross out any alternative with an X in either the first or second box.

Phase Three

Now further simplify your choices by sorting out those that optimize a particular value or ethical concern. Use the third column of boxes and the numbered issues from the warm-up section at the beginning of this exercise.

Reexamine your case and identify the parties directly affected by any decision in the case. List them below.

YOUR LIST OF PARTIES INVOLVED IN THIS CASE BY ID NUMBER

1. _____   2. _____

3. _____   4. _____

5. _____   6. _____

Using the fourth box after each remaining option, indicate by number the party or parties most directly affected by the remaining options.

Finally, rewrite your list rearranging your remaining alternatives. List together in one group all those alternatives affecting a specific person or persons, or those relating to a single ethical concern. You may decide to use both ways of clustering your alternatives. Ask yourself whether two or more options in any cluster can effectively be combined into a single alternative that is more positive and stronger than if the alternatives are considered separately.

YOUR ALTERNATIVES REARRANGED ACCORDING TO ETHICAL PRINCIPLES OR THE PARTIES AFFECTED

Use the lines below to rearrange your alternatives. Attach extra pages as necessary.

_____

_____

_____

_____

_____

_____

_____

_____

8 REACHING AN
OPERATIONAL DECISION

CHAPTER 8 EXERCISE
REACHING AN
OPERATIONAL DECISION*

CASE TITLE

NAME

CLASS

Option Choice

The option I prefer in this case is (circle one): 1 2 3 4

This option is to _____

Phase One

Indicate the three factors or considerations that most influenced your selection of the above option. Indicate the relative importance of these three factors by numbering them 1 (most important), 2, or 3 (least important) in the space after those factors that most influenced your decision.

Economic: Costs to taxpayer, person(s) involved, or health facility affected

_____

Legal: Creating a legal precedent, or a need for new laws or the repeal of laws

_____

*The format for this exercise was adapted from "A Comprehensive Study of the Ethical, Legal, and Social Implications for Advances in Biomedical and Behavioral Research and Technology," a national survey of experts and laypersons conducted by Policy Research, Inc., 2500 North Charles Street, Baltimore, MD 21218, and by the Center for Technology Assessment, New Jersey Institute of Technology, 323 High Street, Newark, NJ 07102.

Social: The effects on society in general, social attitudes, values, priorities, and so on. ____

Political considerations: The effects of this option on our political system and Constitution ____

Personal considerations: The effects of this option on personal values, rights, autonomy, and integrity ____

Religious or ethical factors: Effects of this option in maintaining or hindering moral, religious, or philosophical values you consider important ____

Medical considerations: The consequences of this option on the delivery of health care and on the psychology of health care professionals ____

Technical factors: The possible effects of this option on basic research, on the continued advance of medical science, and on scientists engaged in research and development ____

Other considerations not mentioned above:

_____ ____

_____ ____

_____ ____

Explain below the three factors or considerations that most influenced your decision. Start with your most important factor. Separate each idea or aspect into a single sentence. Be brief and concise. One or two sentences will suffice if your ideas about this particular factor are clearly thought out *before* you start writing.

Most important factor: _____

Explanation: _____

_____

_____

_____

_____

_____

_____

_____

_____

_____

_____

Second most important factor: _____

Explanation: _____

_____

_____

_____

_____

_____

_____

_____

_____

_____

_____

Third most important factor: _____

Explanation: _____

_____

_____

_____

_____

_____

_____

_____

_____

_____

_____

_____

_____

Phase Two

Assume that circumstances in your case allowed you to consult with other persons or parties besides those mentioned in your case. Place a check by those with whom you would have liked to talk.

- Religious, ethical, or philosophical groups _____

- The national professional organizations for physicians, nurses, respiratory or physical therapists, radiologic or medical technologists, or other health care groups _____

- The immediate family of the person involved _____

- The American Bar Association, the hospital or clinical lawyers, the patient's or family's lawyers, a medical malpractice lawyer _____

- A consumer advocacy group pertinent to the case _____

- The courts and judicial system _____

- Other persons in similar situations _____

- The legislative branch of the federal government _____

- The legislative branch of state or local government _____

- A national opinion poll or referendum _____

- Special interest groups such as the American Civil Liberties Union, right to life groups, the National Organization for Women, the National Organization of Non-Parents, the Euthanasia Society of North America, Parents of Adopted Children, and the National Adoptees Rights Association _____

- Private industries, such as pharmaceutical, insurance, or biomedical research corporations _____

- Other individuals or groups as follows:

_____   _____

_____   _____

Among the groups and individuals you checked above, which *one* do you feel is *most important?* _____
What is your reason for this priority?

_____

_____

_____

_____

_____

_____

Phase Three

The circumstances in your case may make outside consultation impossible, but time and circumstances may allow you to consult with one person or group mentioned in your case. If you could talk with anyone mentioned in the case and ask them about missing information, whom would you choose? Who might fill in the gaps in your picture? Whose views and opinions in the case would be most important for you to know in depth?

Indicate below which person you wish to talk with and why as well as what questions you would ask.

_____

_____

_____

_____

_____

_____

_____

_____

_____

_____

Phase Four

Do you believe there is a need for a general public policy to handle this and similar cases? Would we be better off with

• No public policy   _____

• A state policy   _____

• An institutional policy   _____

• A federal nationwide policy   _____

• A community-level policy   _____

   Explain briefly the reasons for your view.

_____

_____

_____

_____

_____

_____

_____

_____

If you do not favor any form of general public policy, can you suggest ways to improve the sharing of ideas between people confronted with decisions similar to those in your case?

_____

_____

_____

_____

_____

_____

_____

_____

_____

Phase Five

Reexamine your case study and select one missing detail or specific piece of information that might alter either the direction or strength of your decision. What is the missing information you would like to have?

_____

_____

_____

_____

Why would this information affect your decision? Could it reverse your decision?

_____

_____

_____

_____

_____

_____

How important is this missing information for you to make the best decision in this case?

• Essential or very important ——

• Helpful but not essential ——

• Needed to confirm my decision ——

• Other (explain in the space below) ——

_____

_____

_____

_____

_____

_____

_____

_____

Outline your thoughts in rough form here before composing your final answers for this exercise.

9 USING AN ALTERNATIVES BALANCE SHEET

CHAPTER 9 EXERCISE
USING AN ALTERNATIVES BALANCE SHEET*

CASE TITLE _____

NAME _____

CLASS _____

FIRST ALTERNATIVE, to _____

Positive consequences. Briefly list below as many positive consequences as you can for this first option. Assign each possible consequence two weights, one for *general importance* (in terms of economics, legal, political, psychological, and other factors) and one for *moral importance.* Use the scale below:

5 = Very important

4 = Important

3 = Worth considering

2 = Of minor importance

1 = Of very minor importance

Your list of positive consequences

	General Weight	Ethical Importance
_____		
_____		
_____		
_____		
_____		

*The format for this exercise is adapted from "A Comprehensive Study of the Ethical, Legal, and Social Implications of Advances in Biomedical and Behavioral Research and Technology," a national survey of experts and laypersons conducted by Policy Research Inc., 2500 North Charles Street, Baltimore, MD 21218, and by the Center for Technology Assessment, New Jersey Institute of Technology, 323 High Street, Newark, NJ 07102.

	General Weight	Ethical Importance
_____		
_____		
_____		
_____		

FIRST ALTERNATIVE, to _____

Negative consequences. Briefly list below as many negative consequences as you can for this first option. Assign each possible consequence a general weight and an ethical weight.

Your list of negative consequences

	General Weight	Ethical Importance
_____		
_____		
_____		
_____		
_____		
_____		
_____		
_____		
_____		

Subtotal of general weights for *positive* consequences _____
Subtotal of general weights for *negative* consequences _____

Subtotal of ethical weights for *positive* consequences   _____
Subtotal of ethical weights for *negative* consequences   _____

Subtract the negative (cost) subtotal from the positive (benefit) subtotal for the general weights and for the ethical weights. If the moral or general positive consequences of this alternative outweigh the negative consequences, you will arrive at a *positive figure*. If the negative consequences of this option are greater, your final total will be a *negative figure*.

What is your final cost/benefit general weight for this option?   _____
What is your final cost/benefit ethical weight for this option?   _____
(Be sure your final figures are either positive or negative.)

SECOND ALTERNATIVE, to _____

Positive consequences. Briefly list below as many positive consequences as you can for this second option. Assign each possible consequence a general weight and an ethical weight.

Your list of positive consequences

	General Weight	Ethical Importance
_____		
_____		
_____		
_____		
_____		
_____		
_____		
_____		
_____		

SECOND ALTERNATIVE, to _____

Negative consequences. Briefly list below as many negative consequences as you can for this second option. Assign each possible consequence a general weight and an ethical weight.

Your list of negative consequences

	General Weight	Ethical Importance
_____		
_____		
_____		
_____		
_____		
_____		
_____		
_____		
_____		

Subtotal of general weights for *positive* consequences   _____
Subtotal of general weights for *negative* consequences   _____

Subtotal of ethical weights for *positive* consequences   _____
Subtotal of ethical weights for *negative* consequences   _____

   Subtract the negative (cost) subtotal from the positive (benefit) subtotal for both the general and ethical weights. If the general or ethical positive consequences of this alternative outweigh the negative consequences, you will arrive at a *positive figure*. If the negative consequences of this option are greater, your final total will be a *negative figure*.

What is your final cost/benefit general weight for this option?   _____
What is your final cost/benefit ethical weight for this option?   _____
(Be sure your final figures are either positive or negative.)

THIRD ALTERNATIVE, to _____

Positive consequences. Briefly list below as many positive consequences as you can for this third option. Assign a general weight and an ethical weight to each possible consequence.

Your list of positive consequences

	General Weight	Ethical Importance
_____		
_____		
_____		
_____		
_____		
_____		
_____		
_____		
_____		

THIRD ALTERNATIVE, to _____

Negative consequences. Briefly list below as many negative consequences as you can for this third option. Assign a general weight and an ethical weight to each possible consequence.

Your list of negative consequences

	General Weight	Ethical Importance
_____		
_____		
_____		
_____		
_____		
_____		
_____		
_____		
_____		

Subtotal of general weights for *positive* consequences _____
Subtotal of general weights for *negative* consequences _____

Subtotal of ethical weights for *positive* consequences _____
Subtotal of ethical weights for *negative* consequences _____

Subtract the negative (cost) subtotal from the positive (benefit) subtotal for both general and ethical weights. If the general or ethical positive consequences of this alternative outweigh the negative consequences, you will arrive at a *positive figure.* If the negative consequences of this option are greater, your final total will be a *negative figure.*

What is your final cost/benefit general weight for this option? _____
What is your final cost/benefit ethical weight for this option? _____
(Be sure your final figures are either positive or negative.)

Alternatives Balance Sheet
Summary

FIRST OPTION

Transfer your subtotals from pages 287, 288, and 290 to this page.

General weight subtotals for positive consequences   _____
                           for negative consequences   _____
Overall, which set of consequences has the greater general weight?
(Circle one.)   POSITIVE   NEGATIVE
By how much?   _____

Ethical weight subtotals for positive consequences   _____
                           for negative consequences   _____
Overall, which set of consequences has the greater ethical weight?
(Circle one.)   POSITIVE   NEGATIVE
By how much?   _____

SECOND OPTION

General weight subtotal for positive consequences   _____
                          for negative consequences   _____
Overall, which set of consequences has the greater general weight?
(Circle one.)   POSITIVE   NEGATIVE
By how much?   _____

Ethical weight subtotals for positive consequences   _____
                           for negative consequences   _____
Overall, which set of consequences has the greater ethical weight?
(Circle one.)   POSITIVE   NEGATIVE
By how much?   _____

THIRD OPTION

General weight subtotals for positive consequences   _____
                           for negative consequences   _____
Overall, which set of consequences has the greater general weight?
(Circle one.)   POSITIVE   NEGATIVE
By how much?   _____

Ethical weight subtotals for positive consequences   _____
                           for negative consequences   _____

Overall, which set of consequences has the greater ethical weight?
(Circle one.)   POSITIVE   NEGATIVE
By how much? _____

Which option has the highest general positive weight?   1   2   3

Which option has the highest ethical positive weight?   1   2   3

Cross-Checking Your Balance Sheet Decision

If you analyzed this same case using the operational decision technique in Chapter 8 or the decisional matrix in Chapter 11, how does your decision arrived at using the balance sheet compare with your other decision in the same case? (Circle one.)   AGREES   DISAGREES
If your two decisions do not agree, how do you explain your conflicting decisions?

_____

_____

_____

_____

_____

Outline your thoughts in rough form here before composing your final answers for this exercise.

10 CREATING A DECISION TREE

CHAPTER 10 EXERCISE
CREATING
A DECISION TREE

_____   _____
CASE TITLE   NAME

                                     _____
                                     CLASS

Phase One

Identify two to four of the most obvious and important decisions or actions you could take in this case. List them below.

_____

_____

_____

_____

_____

_____

_____

On the next two pages create your decision tree. Follow the pattern shown in Figure 10.1 in Part One. Use both pages to sketch out your tree, working from the decision/action node on the far left. (1) Draw a line for each of your two to four decisions or actions from the decision/action node on the far left and end each line at a "chance event" node (a circle) on the first level. (2) Think about what might happen at each first level node and draw lines to the second level. Label each line with its chance event and end each line with another chance node on the second level. (3) Each chance node on the second level must have its two or more subsequent events, with labeled lines going to third level chance event nodes. (4) Repeat this branching process to connect third

continued on page 298

	Subsequent Chance Events	
Original Action	First Level	Second Level

Subsequent Chance Events		
Third Level	Fourth Level	Final Outcome

level nodes with fourth level nodes. (5) Connect fourth level nodes with final outcomes for each line. Remember, some chance events on the first, second, or third level might be final and go directly to the final outcome column on the far right.

Phase Two

Assigned values can now be given to each outcome on the far right of the tree. A zero should be assigned to the ideal final outcome or the least harmful final outcome. Write this assigned value of zero in the appropriate circles on the far right. Decide on a negative value for each of the remaining outcomes and write them in the appropriate circles. The larger your negative number, the more harmful you judge the particular outcome to be (see page 120 in Part One).

Probability figures or estimates can now be added to the chance events on all four levels (see page 122 in Part One).

Check over each item in your tree to make certain you have written in all the necessary assigned values on the far right and probabilities for each chance event.

Phase Three

Start "rolling back" your tree from right to left, following the calculation formula in Chapter 10 of Part One. Start in the lower right hand corner, multiplying the assigned value by its associated probability figure. Repeat to obtain other subtotals and then add the subtotals together to obtain the calculated value. Enter this in a circle with an arrow pointing to the appropriate chance node. Work from bottom to top on each level and from right to left. Take your time and do the calculations step by step, level by level. They are simple and routine but need to be done one at a time. When you finish, each chance node should have a calculated value attached to it.

Check the calculated values for the two to four event nodes on level one next to your initial action/decision node. Which of these calculated values is the lowest, the closest to the ideal outcome? Do you agree that this action or decision is the best one? If so, why? If not, why do you disagree?

_____

_____

_____

_____

_____

Work out your list of assigned values and probabilities (estimated or real) in this space before you start your tree.

11 USING A DECISION MATRIX

CHAPTER 11 EXERCISE
USING A DECISION MATRIX

CASE TITLE

NAME

CLASS

Phase One

In the space below identify your main alternatives.

_____

_____

_____

_____

_____

_____

_____

_____

_____

_____

_____

Phase Two

Circle as many of the following ethical principles as are involved in this case.

1. Autonomy

2. Veracity

301

3. Nonmaleficence

4. Beneficence

5. Confidentiality

6. Justice

List the ethical values or criteria derived from or dependent on these moral principles as they apply to this case. (See page 55.)

_____

_____

_____

_____

_____

_____

_____

_____

_____

_____

_____

_____

Add to this list of ethical values any nonmoral consequences or values you believe should be considered in your decision process.

_____

_____

_____

_____

_____

_____

In the space below, rearrange your values in a ranking from the most important at the top of your list to the least important at the bottom. Assign each value an order number, indicating its relative importance to you. Obtain your total and divide each value's order number by this total to obtain its weighting factor. Enter all numerical data in the table below. Refer to pages 132–133 in Part One if you need to refresh your memory of how this is done.

Value	Order Number	Weighting Factor
TOTAL		

Phases Three and Four

Use the data in the table above to construct your decision matrix (Exercise Fig. 11.1) as follows:

1. Across the top, list your selection values or criteria, both ethical and non-moral. Start with the selection value you assigned the highest order number, on the left, and end with the criterion of the lowest order, on the right.

2. List your alternatives down the left side.

3. Transfer the weighting factor for each selection value to the square just below the appropriate value and above the columns of boxes with diagonals.

4. Assign each alternative a rating factor on a scale of 10 (highest) to 1 (lowest). Enter each rating factor in the shaded *upper half* of each box for each combination of value and alternative. You should have a rating factor for each box in your chart.

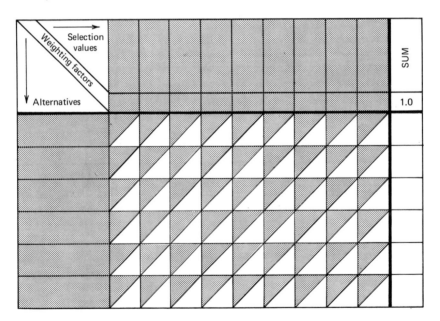

EXERCISE FIGURE 11.1 *Decision matrix form with spaces for entering information on (1) alternatives, (2) selection values for the alternatives, (3) weighting factors, and (4) the assigned rating factor. See instructions in the exercises for filling in these shaded areas.*

(Format from Hill, P., et al. *Making Decisions: A Multidisciplinary Introduction.* Reading, MA: Addison-Wesley, 1978, pp. 124–125. Reprinted with permission.)

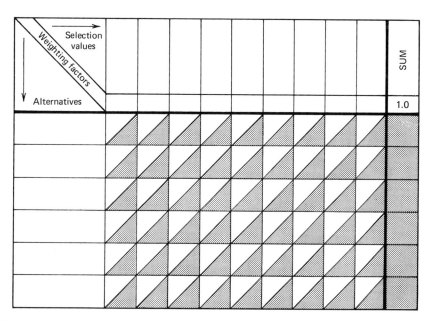

EXERCISE FIGURE 11.2 *Decision matrix form with spaces for entering information on products obtained from multiplying each combination of rating factor and weighting factor. These products should be entered in the appropriate shaded lower half of each box. The four sets of data should be filled in from Figure 11.1 before completing the sums on the far right.*

(Format from Hill, P., et al. *Making Decisions: A Multidisciplinary Introduction.* Reading, MA: Addison-Wesley, 1978, pp. 124–125. Reprinted with permission.)

Phase Five

Next, for each combination of alternative and selection value, multiply the value's weighting factor by the rating factor you assigned for that combination. This will give you a product that you can enter in the lower shaded half of the appropriate square (Exercise Fig. 11.2). Complete this multiplication process for each combination of rating factor and weighting factor.

Now add all the products in the lower half of all the boxes opposite each alternative. Enter the total for each alternative in the appropriate box at the far right under *Sum.*

Finally, determine which alternative has the highest confidence level among the sums on the far right. If you have been conscientious and thorough with your determination of ethical principles and selection values involved in this case, your listing of alternatives, and your assigning of weighting and rating factors, the alternative with the highest confidence level on the far right should be your most ethical alternative.

12 COPING WITH THE LEAST DESIRABLE OPTION

CHAPTER 12 EXERCISE
COPING WITH THE LEAST
DESIRABLE OPTION*

CASE TITLE

NAME

CLASS

Circle the alternative you prefer in this case: 1 2 3 4. Write out the alternative: _____

_____

Circle the option you are *most opposed to:* 1 2 3 4. Write out the option:

_____

_____

If the option you are most opposed to is implemented by an ethics committee or a supervisor's decision, and you do not withdraw from the case, you must deal with the negative consequences of this least desirable alternative. This may mean doing whatever you can to minimize the harm that you anticipate.

First, identify what you believe are the three most negative consequences of this least desirable alternative. This can be done in the space at the top of the next several pages. Then for each of the three negative consequences, identify two or three groups you believe would be most affected by these consequences. These affected parties may differ for the three negative consequences you iden-

*The format for this exercise is adapted from "A Comprehensive Study of the Ethical, Legal, and Social Implications of Advances in Biomedical and Behavioral Research and Technology," conducted by Policy Research, Inc., 2500 North Charles Street, Baltimore, MD 21218, and by the Center for Technology Assessment, New Jersey Institute of Technology, 323 High Street, Newark, NJ 07102.

tify. Use the list below as a guide, but list the parties affected under each of your negative consequences on the next few pages.

Ethnic or racial minorities

Illegal aliens

People in other countries

Urban Americans

Rural Americans

Low-income persons

Middle-income persons

Wealthy persons

Children under 18

Adults ages 18 to 35

Adults ages 36 to 60

Adults over 60

College-educated persons

High school graduates

Persons with elementary school education only

Healthy persons

Acutely ill persons

Chronically ill persons

Institutionalized persons

Prison inmates

Unemployed welfare recipients

Biomedical researchers

Private industry

Insurance companies

Pharmaceutical companies

Government

Health care professionals

Other (specify)

The most significant negative consequence I anticipate if my least desirable alternative is implemented is

_____

_____

_____

_____

_____

The groups I feel would suffer most from this prime consequence are

1. _____

2. _____

3. _____

In the space below describe in detail this major negative consequence. Organize your description to include the specific effects on the groups you listed above. Number your brief statements.

_____

_____

_____

_____

_____

_____

_____

_____

_____

_____

_____

_____

The second most significant negative consequence I anticipate if my least desirable alternative is implemented is

_____

_____

_____

_____

_____

The groups I feel would suffer most from this second negative consequence are

1. _____

2. _____

3. _____

In the space below describe in detail this second negative consequence. Organize your description to include the specific effects on the groups you listed above. Number your statements.

_____

_____

_____

_____

_____

_____

_____

_____

_____

_____

_____

_____

The third most significant negative consequence I anticipate if my least desirable option is implemented is

_____

_____

_____

_____

The groups I feel would suffer most from this third negative consequence are

1. _____

2. _____

3. _____

In the space below describe in detail this third negative consequence. Organize your description to include the specific effects on the groups you listed above. Number your statements.

_____

_____

_____

_____

_____

_____

_____

_____

_____

_____

_____

_____

_____

_____

Assume that the alternative you think is most unethical and least desirable is implemented. As the chief critic of this alternative you are given the task of designing specific steps to reduce the harm. What specific policies, laws, guidelines, regulations, or other action would you recommend to ameliorate the situation? You can approach this task in at least two ways. First, you might figure out a way to minimize the negative consequence you anticipate. Second, you might devise ways to compensate those who actually suffer harm from this alternative.

On this page, focus on your first negative consequence. Be concise and specific. Describe what should or might be done to cope with the most significant negative consequence.

_____

_____

_____

_____

_____

_____

_____

_____

_____

_____

_____

_____

_____

_____

_____

_____

_____

_____

On this last page, focus on ameliorating the situation in terms of your second most harmful consequence.

_____

_____

_____

_____

_____

_____

_____

_____

_____

_____

_____

_____

_____

_____

_____

_____

_____

_____

_____

_____

_____

_____

_____

_____

_____

CHAPTER 13 EXERCISE
ANALYZING THE EFFECTS
OF MOTIVATIONS

CASE TITLE

NAME

CLASS

Phase One

Identify the three or four main parties in this case:

• The central person _____

• The second main party _____

• The third main party _____

• The fourth main party _____

Think over the options for your case and decide on one alternative to use in this exercise. All of your motives will center around this one option. The motives you find in your case and the ones you create to complete the possibilities will all be motives related to the one option you select as a focus. Write this option on the line below.

_____

Phase Two

Read your case through slowly two or three times. Look for motives the people in the case express or motives that are attributed to them by others. Decide whether each motive is "altruistic," "hedonistic/egotistic," or "pragmatic/utilitarian." Name the person in the case. Then write the actual motives in the appropriate spaces below. Mark these with an asterisk.

Next, create motives for each of the persons to fill in the blanks. Some motives you think of may not fit into one of the three categories of altruistic, hedonistic, or pragmatic. You can write these motives in the fourth space at the end of each section of motives for the person concerned.

The central person in this case: _____

An altruistic motive for this person

_____

_____

_____

_____

A hedonistic motive for this person

_____

_____

_____

_____

A pragmatic motive for this person

_____

_____

_____

_____

A motive that does not fit any of the above categories

_____

_____

_____

_____

_____

_____

The second person in this case: _____

An altruistic motive for this person

_____

_____

_____

_____

A hedonistic motive for this person

_____

_____

_____

_____

A pragmatic motive for this person

_____

_____

_____

_____

A motive that does not fit any of the above categories

_____

_____

_____

_____

The third person in this case: _____

An altruistic motive for this person

_____

_____

_____

_____

A hedonistic motive for this person

_____

_____

_____

_____

A pragmatic motive for this person

_____

_____

_____

_____

A motive that does not fit any of the above categories

_____

_____

_____

_____

_____

The fourth person in this case: _____

An altruistic motive for this person

_____

_____

_____

A hedonistic motive for this person

_____

_____

_____

_____

A pragmatic motive for this person

_____

_____

_____

_____

A motive that does not fit the above categories

_____

_____

_____

_____

_____

_____

Phase Three

How does your awareness of these motives affect your selection of the most ethical option in this case?

_____

_____

_____

_____

_____

_____

_____

_____

_____

_____

_____

What particular motive of one person in the case would lead you to seriously consider changing your original decision of the most ethical option?

_____

_____

_____

_____

_____

_____

_____

_____

_____

_____

In your list, can you find a combination of several motives for two or more different persons that when considered together might lead you to make a different decision than you were originally inclined toward?

_____

_____

_____

_____

_____

_____

_____

_____

_____

_____

_____

Outline your thoughts in rough form here before composing your final answers for this exercise.

CHAPTER 14 EXERCISE
ANALYZING THE IMPACT
OF PRESENTATION MODES

CASE TITLE

NAME

CLASS

Phase One

Using either the case presented by the "Ole Nincompoop" or another case assigned by the instructor, make a list of all the emotionally biased and shock-value words, phrases, and ideas expressed in the case. If a film or videotape was used in the presentation, list all the visual images or techniques that had a strong emotional impact on you.

_____

_____

_____

_____

_____

_____

_____

_____

_____

_____

_____

_____

Phase Two

Rewrite your case presentation in the space below. (Type it if you can.) If you wish, reverse the bias and rewrite the presentation with a similarly strong but opposite bias. Or, if you prefer, use the same facts and rewrite them in a case that poses the ethical issue of your assigned case but in an unbiased, objective way. If a case other than the "Ole Nincompoop" is assigned and the written/oral presentation was clinically and not emotionally presented, rewrite it using strong emotional and biased language in favor of a definite position or solution. If a film was used, offer some suggestions on how the emotional impact of the film might be reversed or neutralized.

Use this space for continuing your rewrite and suggestions for new images.

In the second excerpt, "Ole Nincompoop" offers his ideas on why this ethical dilemma is so common. Briefly state your views on his analysis. Do you agree or disagree with his analysis? If you use a different case, what do you believe is the main cause of the problem?

_____

_____

_____

_____

_____

_____

_____

Finally, under the three headings below, list your criteria for examples of situations in which you believe it would be ethically appropriate or inappropriate to employ the medical procedure involved in your case.

Procedure Is Totally Inappropriate and Unethical When:	*Procedure Is Clearly Appropriate and Ethical When:*	*Situations in Which It Is Unclear What Is Most Ethical and Appropriate Exist When:*

Outline your thoughts in rough form here before composing your final answers for this exercise.

CHAPTER 15 EXERCISE
MAKING CONSENSUS OR COMMITTEE DECISIONS

CASE TITLE

NAME

CLASS

Phase One

List the alternatives identified by the group or committee.

_____

_____

_____

_____

_____

_____

_____

_____

_____

_____

_____

_____

_____

_____

Identify by number the options selected for discussion from the list above and include the names of the students assigned or volunteering as advocates to explain and defend the alternatives selected.

Option 1: _____

_____

Option 2: _____

_____

Option 3: _____

_____

Option 4: _____

_____

Option 5: _____

_____

Option 6: _____

_____

Circle the vote that constitutes a deciding faction.

51% majority   Simple plurality

Majority of two-thirds   Plurality over ___%

75% majority

The committee's decision was to _____

_____

_____

My personal preference was to _____

_____

_____

_____

_____

Phase Two

Briefly evaluate the decision-making skills exercised by the members of your committee. To what extent did they demonstrate specific skills based on the previous exercises? Can you cite specific examples?

_____

_____

_____

_____

_____

_____

_____

_____

_____

How comfortable are you with the decision reached by your committee? On what specific issues are you in disagreement with the committee decision? How might you use the technique of coping with the least desirable option (Chapter 12) to reduce some of your discomfort?

_____

_____

_____

_____

_____

_____

_____

_____

_____

_____

_____

CHAPTER 16 EXERCISE
CREATING A PROFILE
FOR PERSONHOOD

NAME _____

CLASS _____

Phase One

Whatever your own personal position, assume for the moment the position of an advocate of a fixed philosophy of the world. This means that there is some specific temporal point in development at which the human organism becomes fully a person, endowed with all the rights and bearing all the responsibilities we commonly attribute to a person. Before that point in time, the organism is not a person. Beyond that point, it possesses inalienable human rights equal to those possessed by any other person. At a second specific time, the moment of death, the person ceases to exist. Recall Figure 1.1 and remember that the holder of this philosophical position sees things as either all or nothing, as either existing fully or not at all.

You can use either end of the human lifespan. Several different starting points are suggested early in Chapter 16. Define your starting or end point. Think through your arguments carefully beforehand. Then write a brief exposition and defense of your starting or end point in the space below.

_____

_____

_____

_____

_____

_____

_____

333

_____

_____

_____

_____

_____

_____

_____

_____

_____

_____

_____

_____

The process view of personhood, which underlies the tentative profile pro-posed by Joseph Fletcher, focuses on the qualities that mark our becoming and our ceasing to be persons. Select one or more qualities of personhood from Fletcher's list, summarized in this exercise. You can refer to Fletcher's expla-nation in the chapter, but use your own views and arguments. You may want to adopt one of the positions of the commentators who objected to Fletcher's use of neocortical activity as the single central criterion.

Think through your exposition and defense of the criterion or criteria you selected carefully before writing it in the space below.

_____

_____

_____

_____

_____

_____

_____

_____

_____

_____

_____

_____

_____

_____

_____

_____

_____

_____

_____

_____

_____

_____

_____

_____

_____

_____

Phase Two

Reexamine Fletcher's indicators of personhood below in terms of your own views. Then answer the four questions he asks in the conclusion of his paper.

1. Pick out one or more cardinal indicators that you believe are absolutely essential and central to the nature of our personhood. Mark these in the first column of the table on page 336.

2. Choose among the remaining qualities or characteristics that you believe are important as optimal indicators. These are qualities that are important but not essential in our definition of personhood. Indicate these in the second column.

3. Which factors can be eliminated, in part or in whole, from our basic definition of personhood without lowering individuals below the personal line? Cross these out altogether.

4. Finally, in the three columns on the right, rank the optimal qualities of personhood in terms of their priority for you. This ranking can be done on the basis you used in Chapters 4, 9, and 11. Under the first subhead, give an order number to each of the optimal factors. You may decide to give two or more factors the same order number to indicate their parity. Under the second subhead, divide the order number by the total (ON/T). Enter the result of this division for each indicator under the third subhead as the final weighting factor (WF) for that criterion.

Weighting the Indicators of Personhood: A Tentative Ranking

Criteria	Cardinal Factor(s)	Optimal Factors	Weighting		
			Order No.	ON/T	WF
Positive					
Minimal intelligence					
Self-awareness					
Self-control					
A sense of time					
A sense of futurity					
A sense of the past					
Ability to relate interpersonally					
Concern for others					
Communication					
Control of life					
Curiosity					
Changeability					
Idiosyncrasy					
Neocortical function					
Negative					
Not non- or anti-artificial					
Not essentially parental					
Not essentially sexual					
Not a bundle of rights					
Not a worshiper					
			TOTAL:		

What basic problems do you see for modern medicine in trying to use a fixed philosophy definition of personhood?

_____

_____

_____

_____

_____

_____

_____

_____

_____

_____

What basic problems do you see for modern medicine in trying to apply a process definition of personhood?

_____

_____

_____

_____

_____

_____

_____

_____

_____

_____

INDEX OF CASE STUDIES
AND ETHICAL ISSUES

Since this worktext focuses on the elements and processes of making ethical decisions, our case studies are somewhat of a side issue. The cases are frankly too brief and incomplete to qualify as professional case studies or as clinical presentations. Rather, their function is to serve as the grist in applying the elements and various techniques of making ethical decisions. The lists below of the issues and cases dealt with in the individual chapters are provided as aids in cross-reference.

Issues and Cases Listed by Chapter

Issues and Cases Listed by Topics

INSTANT REFERENCE KEY

Match the tabs to quickly locate chapters and their corresponding exercises.

PART ONE: CHAPTERS

1 TWO WORLD VIEWS AND TWO ASSOCIATED VALUE SYSTEMS

2 THREE MODELS OF MORAL DEVELOPMENT

3 IDENTIFYING ETHICAL PRINCIPLES

4 IDENTIFYING AND WEIGHTING ETHICAL RULES

5 DECISIONS IN TRIAGE SITUATIONS

6 THE SOCIAL CONTRACT BETWEEN PATIENT AND HEALTH CARE WORKER

7 IDENTIFYING AND SORTING ALTERNATIVE SOLUTIONS

8 THE OPERATIONAL DECISION TECHNIQUE

9 COSTS AND BENEFITS OF AN ALTERNATIVES BALANCE SHEET

10 THE DECISION TREE TECHNIQUE

11 THE DECISION MATRIX TECHNIQUE

12 A TECHNIQUE FOR COPING WITH THE LEAST DESIRABLE OPTION

13 ASCERTAINING THE EFFECTS OF MOTIVATIONS ON DECISIONS

14 EXAMINING THE IMPACT OF MODES OF PRESENTATION

15 CONSENSUS DECISIONS FOR PUBLIC POLICIES

16 THE ULTIMATE QUESTION: WHO IS A PERSON, AND WHY?

CONCLUSION: A SYNTHESIS OF DECISION-MAKING METHODS

PART TWO: EXERCISES

1 DUTY-ORIENTED AND CONSEQUENCE-ORIENTED THINKING

2 GENDER-RELATED MORAL THINKING

3 IDENTIFYING ETHICAL PRINCIPLES

4 IDENTIFYING AND WEIGHTING ETHICAL RULES

5 MAKING TRIAGE DECISIONS

6 ANALYZING THE HEALTH CARE SOCIAL CONTRACT

7 IDENTIFYING AND SORTING ALTERNATIVES

8 REACHING AN OPERATIONAL DECISION

9 USING AN ALTERNATIVES BALANCE SHEET

10 CREATING A DECISION TREE

11 USING A DECISION MATRIX

12 COPING WITH THE LEAST DESIRABLE OPTION

13 ANALYZING THE EFFECTS OF MOTIVATIONS

14 ANALYZING THE IMPACT OF PRESENTATION MODES

15 MAKING CONSENSUS OR COMMITTEE DECISIONS

16 CREATING A PROFILE FOR PERSONHOOD

INDEX OF CASE STUDIES AND ETHICAL ISSUES